HOSPITAL POLICY
IN THE
UNITED KINGDOM

HOSPITAL POLICY
IN THE
UNITED KINGDOM
Its Development, Its Future

Anthony Harrison and Sally Prentice

Transaction Publishers
New Brunswick (U.S.A.) and London (U.K.)

This book is printed on acid-free paper that meets the American National Standard for Permanence of Paper for Printed Library Materials.

Library of Congress Catalog Number: 97-230
ISBN: 1-56000-978-0
Printed in the United States of America

Library of Congress Cataloging-in-Publication Data

Harrison, Anthony.
    Hospital policy in the United Kingdom : its development, its future / Anthony Harrison and Sally Prentice.
        p. cm.
    Originally published: Acute futures. London : King's Fund. c1996.
Includes bibliographical references and index.
ISBN 1-56000-978-0 (pbk. : alk. paper)
1. Hospitals—Great Britain—Planning. 2. Medical policy—Great Britain.
I. Prentice, Sally. II. Harrison, Anthony Acute Futures. III. Title.
    [DNLM: 1. Hospital Planning—Great Britain. 2. Policy Making—Great Britain. WX 140 H318h 1996a]
RA986.H37   1997
362.1'1'0941—dc21
DNLM/DLC
for Library of Congress   97-230
                                                                                 CIP

Contents

Preface

During the time this study has been in preparation, a number of reports have been published advocating changes in the way hospital services are organised and provided. In some cases, particular 'solutions' have been proposed such as massive superhospitals serving 2 million people. Others, in contrast, argue for massive switches away from hospitals into other forms of care.

Readers looking for 'solutions', blueprints or specific proposals of this kind will be disappointed. What we have aimed to provide is a source of reference and reflection for those who are concerned with the planning of hospitals themselves or who are, perhaps by virtue of their role as purchasers, concerned with the health care delivery system as a whole.

Those faced with these difficult tasks face many challenges, not least among them the lack of any tradition in this country of study of the hospital and hospital policy. This absence does not reflect a lack of concern about hospital services, but rather a failure on the one hand to analyse the institution as a whole, as opposed to the individual specialty or function, and on the other to make explicit the assumptions that have guided policy in practice. As a result, much of what is known or believed to be the case is not written down and hence made subject to critical assessment. A further consequence is that what is not known is not apparent either. Although we hope that the range of empirical material we draw on here will be helpful, we also hope that this report will not be judged by that alone. For what we have tried to do is develop a structure of analysis which was originally set out in the 1960s by those then responsible for hospital policy and which has proved its durability by retaining its relevance to the present day.

That structure, focusing on quality of care, access and costs of provision, provides not only a way of setting out the basic policy issues which hospital planners have to tackle, but also a framework for marshalling the available empirical evidence. It also creates 'slots' for evidence which as yet does not exist by identifying the knowledge we would like to have.

The 1960s framework is not infinitely durable. New technology particularly in IT has been developed which allows 'access at a distance' in a way undreamed of 30 years ago. But in its essentials it still holds. What therefore we have attempted to do is refine and elaborate it and then set what evidence we have been able to find within it. As more comes to hand, its significance should be all the clearer for finding a 'slot' within an explicit structure. That, at least, is our hope.

The report draws on a wide range of published sources, our debt to which will be found at the end of this volume. However, we have been helped in the course of this study by a large number of people in the course of visits to particular hospitals, meetings with representatives of professional organisations or groups representing patients, officials in the Department of Health and the Audit Commission, as well as colleagues from all parts of the King's Fund, those within Information Resources for their tracking down of material on our behalf. As is is customary, we ascribe all the errors and omissions to ourselves.

We are grateful for comments received from Keith Willett at the John Radcliffe Hospital, Tony Redmond at the North Staffordshire Trauma Centre and Philip Hadridge in the NHS Management Executive Anglia and Oxford Office. Jeremy Jones suggested the procedures selected in Chapter 4. We are also grateful to Jackie Mallender for her critical and constructive comments and to the late Peter Dixon, Public Health Director at West Berkshire, for helpful discussion early on in this project. We also owe a particular debt to Jill Tyler, then working with the National Case Mix Office, for carrying out the data analysis used in Chapter 2 and elsewhere in this report and to Phil Anthony, Research Director at the Office, for encouraging and facilitating the work.

Anthony Harrison
Sally Prentice

CHAPTER I

The development of hospital policy

When the National Health Service (NHS) was established, it inherited a collection of hospital assets which no national health authority would have invested in, had one existed before the war. Surveys both before and after the Second World War identified large variations between different parts of the country in the quality and the quantity of provision. A third of consultant staff were located in London and some parts of the country, such as what is now the Anglia and Oxford Region, had virtually none. In other areas, facilities were duplicated as a result of parallel developments by local authorities and voluntary bodies.

Economic difficulties in the immediate post-war period ruled out any immediate rationalisation and modernisation. It was not until the 1960s that a serious attempt was made to reshape those assets into a national system of hospital provision. The 1962 Hospital Plan for England and Wales, and its counterparts for the other parts of the UK, represented the first national attempt to provide an acceptable standard of hospital services across the country as a whole. According to Webster (1988):

> The major innovation of the National Health Service was its state-owned and exchequer-funded hospital service. For the first time comprehensive hospital and consultant care was made available to all, and without imposition of direct charges. Inadequacy of specialist services was the most glaring defect of the inter-war system of medical care. Alleviation of this defect was a primary incentive for the first tentative moves towards a national hospital plan. (p 257)

The aim of the Plan (Ministry of Health, 1962) was:

> to give to the hospital service of England and Wales both the physical equipment and also the pattern and setting which will everywhere place the most modern treatment at the service of patients and enable the staffs who care for them to exercise their skill and devotion under the best conditions. (p iii)

The Plan proposed that each district of around 100–150,000 people should have a hospital – known then, as now, as a district general hospital or DGH – in which all but a few specialties – radiotherapy, neurosurgery and plastic surgery which would be provided at only a few sites – were represented. Within this vision of the future, small hospitals were to be retained, particularly in less densely settled parts of the country, where distances to the nearest district general hospital would be too great.

Thus the hospital service on this model would be in three tiers, with the vast majority of work done in the middle one, the district general hospital. The 'higher' tier would contain more specialised facilities, and obtain patients by onward referral from DGHs: most research and teaching would be carried out in such referral institutions which would normally also provide DGH services as well. The lower tier would provide a very limited range of facilities, such as care for the elderly.

After 1962, a number of planning documents appeared in which different views were put forward as to the desirable size of catchment area for a district general hospital on the one hand, and the role of the smaller hospital on the other. In 1969, the Bonham-Carter Report *The Functions of the District General Hospital* (DHSS, 1969) reaffirmed the notion of a general hospital, dismissing the development of separate hospitals for children, women, accidents or orthopaedics. It argued that the 1962 Plan had understated the case for concentrating medical resources and hence proposed that the average hospital size should be much bigger. Whereas the 1962 Plan had proposed catchment populations of some 100–150,000, the Committee suggested that these figures might be doubled. Given the lengths of inpatient stay then current, that meant hospitals might contain some 1,500 beds. That view did not win general support; the Bonham-Carter Report had only a modest impact on the physical size of hospitals. Few hospitals with more than 1,000 beds were ever built.

Although the 1962 Plan and the Bonham-Carter Report endorsed the notion of general hospitals providing a comprehensive service, they also allowed a role, if a modest one, to other kinds of hospital. As the Plan put it:

> *But many small hospitals will still be needed. Some will be retained as maternity units, though any additional provision will nearly always be at the district general hospital. Others will provide long-stay geriatric units. Others again, where a local population is remote or inaccessible, or where isolated towns receive an exceptional seasonal influx of visitors, will continue to admit medical emergencies which do not require specialist facilities. Finally, though this is not indicated in detail in the plan, many small hospitals where no beds, or at least no acute beds, need eventually be retained will be suitable for providing out patient services. (para 2.5)*

Later reports continued to promote the role of the small hospital. Circular DS 85/75 (Department of Health, 1975) proposed that most hospital services should be based on general and community hospitals: the latter were to have between 50 and 150 beds – much larger than most of the existing small institutions – and were to be run by general practitioners under the general oversight of consultants. The Royal Commission on the NHS (DHSS, 1979) suggested that up to one quarter of all inpatient beds might be in community hospitals.

A year later, a Consultation Document, *The Future of Hospital Provision in England* (DHSS, 1980) reaffirmed the validity of the district general hospital, while suggesting that some such institutions were too large:

> *Experience has shown that a large degree of concentration on a single site may in itself have serious disadvantages. Communications of all kinds within the hospital become more complex and difficult, as does management. Patients and relatives, as well as staff, find the hospital too impersonal. It often suffers from physical disadvantages and the need to provide air-conditioning, with high energy requirements. (p 10)*

It then went on to point to other disadvantages:

> *Steep rises in motoring costs means that travel to hospital is more expensive for patients, staff and visitors. Ambulances and other forms of hospital transport all cost more to run. Public transport costs more. And in rural districts it is not as comprehensive, nor as frequent, as it used to be – an important factor for many elderly patients and mothers with young children. (p 11)*

Accordingly, it proposed that the policy of concentration should be changed by placing less emphasis on the centralisation of services in very large hospitals and hence allowing a wider range of local facilities to be retained. It argued that small or medium-sized hospitals would continue to have a role, partly on access grounds both for patients and staff and partly to relieve pressures on the main hospital which, it argued, might become too large and hard to manage if all services were concentrated on one site.

Since 1980, the Government has published no general statement about what the form and content of district general hospitals should be, despite the scale of its commitment to building or refurbishing the existing stock. It has been left to Regional Health Authorities to form their own strategies in the light of the resources likely to be available to them and to guide district health authorities through their control over capital allocations.

Table 1.1   Hospital planning: key dates and publications

1962   Hospital Plan for England and Wales
1966   Revision of the Hospital Plan for England and Wales
1969   The Functions of the District General Hospital (Bonham-Carter Report)
1975   Departmental Circular: Community Hospitals: their role and development in the NHS
       DS 85/75 Review of Health Services and Resources: Planning Tasks for 1975/76
1977   Priorities for Health and Personal Social Services: The Way Forward
1979   Report of the Royal Commission on the NHS
1980   DHSS Consultation Document: Hospital Services: The Future Pattern of Hospital Provision in England

The current pattern of hospital provision is far from conforming to the 1962 blueprint: there is a smaller number of beds doing more work as medical technology has allowed more work to be done in fewer beds than was then envisaged. As a result, although there are many fewer hospitals now than there were then, the size of district general hospitals measured in terms of beds has not risen.

Economic factors, too, have influenced the way that the Plan was implemented. The so-called IMF crisis in the mid-1970s led to major cutbacks in the hospital building programme and the 1980 Consultation Document made it clear that planning had to proceed on a piecemeal basis. To assist with this, the Department developed the nucleus hospital modular design which allowed capacity to be added in incremental but compatible stages. Furthermore, the Consultation Document recognised that in practice the district services might be spread over more than one site since the capital funds to unify them might not be available. In this way, the district general hospital became, and in some way remains, an organisational concept applied over separate sites rather than a single cluster of related clinical activity.

Nevertheless, despite the impact of economic and technological factors, the district general hospital has remained the guiding idea for hospital development up to the present day. Although opinions have altered as to how large, and precisely what its range of activities should be, the idea of a single hospital or, in the case of split sites, a single management unit, serving the majority of the health needs of a district – or part of one in some parts of the country – has remained influential, both in plans for new or replacement hospitals, as well as plans for the configuration of existing facilities. All districts in England contain a DGH and in Wales only rural Powys relies on services provided outside its own district for acute hospital care.

Despite the support offered in the various official reports listed in Table 1.1, the small hospital has not, except in a few parts of the country, retained or achieved the position in the health care system envisaged for it in the 1970s. Community hospitals are typically much smaller but carry out a similar range of functions to those envisaged in the 1970s: see Table 1.2. In addition, there were, as late as 1989, a large number of small hospitals caring for particular care groups: see Table 1.3. Since then, following the creation of trusts, official figures do not identify individual hospital sites. But in May 1995, the Shadow Secretary of State for Health, Margaret Beckett, drawing on figures obtained by the House of Commons Research Division, revealed that 245 hospitals had been closed between 1990 and 1994: see Table 1.4. Most of these were institutions specialising in the care of particular groups of patients. During the same period, a handful of new hospitals were opened, most replacing or modernising existing facilities.

Table 1.2   Comparison of current provision with the original DHSS guidance HSC(IS)75

1975	1985
Designated community hospitals	Official designation not often made
50–150 beds	Up to 50 beds
Mainly GP community beds with beds for the elderly. Beds only exceptionally provided for other specialties	Between 10 and 28 GP community beds, with provision for other specialties
Respite care	Respite care
Day hospital	Few have day hospitals
Consultant outpatient clinics	Consultant outpatient clinics
Minor casualty	Minor casualty
No operating theatre	Most have full operating theatre
Diagnostic services	Diagnostic services
Health centre on site, or associated	Few health centres on site

Source: Tucker (1987)

Table 1.3   Small NHS hospitals, England 1989/90

Total	1061
Mental handicap	459
Mental illness	113
Geriatric medicine	123
General practice	147
Others	219

Source: Higgins (1993)

Table 1.4   Hospital closures, England 1990–1994

Type of Hospital	Number Closed
Total	245
Acute	60
Psychiatric	85
Geriatric	60
Maternity	14
Other	26

Source: Labour Party Press Release

As Table 1.5 shows, the number of small hospitals has fallen, as has the number of very large units, while numbers in the middle ranges have risen in absolute terms and as a proportion of the total. According to Higgins (1993), the events of the 1980s marginalised the role of the small hospital so while a number of reports appeared on what their role might be, no national level response has been forthcoming. Instead Regions have gone their own way: some, particularly the more rural ones, aiming to retain smaller hospitals, others seeking to close down such units and consolidate all activities into central sites. As a result, some areas of the country retain a network of small hospitals carrying out some of the functions to be found elsewhere in general hospitals; in others, they have virtually disappeared.

At the other end of the scale, some services such as neurosurgery and plastic surgery are only available in a few hospitals, so patients needing them must travel outside their district. Typically, they are to be found in teaching hospitals, but elsewhere energetic physicians have been able to develop specialised services within DGHs. In a few instances, the so-called supra-regional services, the Department of Health has intervened to ensure their availability by

Table 1.5   Number of non-psychiatric hospitals: England

	1959	1979	1989/90
Total	2,138	1,609	1,185
Up to 50 beds	912	601	421
21–250	925	705	495
251-500	216	190	162
501-1,000	76	103	105
Over 1,000	9	10	3

Source: Health and Personal Social Statistics, various years

channelling finances directly to them. The criteria for obtaining this privileged financial status were set out in Health Circular (83)36 as follows:

> *. . . services which, in order to be economically viable or clinically effective, need to be provided for a population substantially larger than that of any one Region.*

The current supra-regional specialties are shown in Table 1.6.

Table 1.6   Supra-regional specialties

Choriocarninoma
Cranofacial
Fulminate Liver
Heart Transplantation
Liver Transplantation
Neonatal and Infant Cardiac Surgery
Paediatric Liver
Endoprosthetic Replacement for Primary Bone Tumour
Proton Therapy for Large Uveal Melanomas
Psychiatric Services for Deaf People
Retinoblastoma
Severe Combined Immunodeficiency and Related Disorders

Source: House of Commons Health Committee, Memorandum from the Department of Health on Public Expenditure on Health & Social Services, Session 1993/94, HC617.

Thus the English hospital system is a hierarchical system, but it is not a uniform one. The differences to be found between different parts of the country stem partly from geography and the accidents of history. They also stem from a lack of clarity as to the appropriate division of roles between the different tiers. For example, although plans for a national system of cancer care were formulated before the foundation of the NHS, similar proposals for a hierarchical system of care were put forward by an expert committee in 1995 in the light of evidence that patients were not being referred to the specialist services their needs required. Similarly, a report by the Clinical Services Advisory Committee (1994) presented evidence that access to specialist heart surgery varied widely between different parts of the country. In these and other services for which DGHs may not be the appropriate place of care, there has been no national policy to ensure a similar level of availability throughout the country. The same is true for services within DGHs. A recent study of the provision of intensive care (Metcalfe and McPherson, 1995) found wide variations in its availability as well as in the form of provision, ie the balance between intensive and high-dependency care.

The position is only slightly clearer as to what part the hospital should play in the health care system as a whole. The 1962 Plan recognised that the role of the hospital should be analysed within a wider context:

> *In drawing up the hospital plan, it has been assumed that the first concern of the health and welfare services will continue to be to forestall illness and disability by preventive measures; and that where illness and disability nevertheless occurs, the aim will be to provide care at home and in the community for all who do not require the special types of diagnosis and treatment which only the hospital can provide. (para 31)*

Successive official statements have continued to propose a reduction in the acute hospital's role. The Royal Commission, reporting at the end of the 1970s, stated that 'the emphasis on acute services and high technology is being challenged and more thought is being given to the non-acute sector'. *The Way Ahead* (DHSS, 1977) explicitly suggested that acute services should be cut back to allow the so-called Cinderella services to be developed. But the means and the will to implement this policy proved insufficient. Hospital-based acute services continued to expand throughout the 1980s and into the 1990s, absorbing a higher proportion of the medical workforce and maintaining its share of a rising health budget; see Tables 1.7 and 1.8.

Table 1.7 Medical staffing, England

	1976	1981	1986	1991
Hospital	29,357	33,941	36,305	41,427
GPs	21,975	24,359	26,529	27,888

Notes: Hospital staff figures exclude locums and are full-time equivalents
Source: Health & Personal Social Service Statistics, various years

Table 1.8 Acute care growth and budget share (1992/93 prices), England

	1981/82	1992/93
Total Spend (£m)	9,888	12,185
Share of Total Hospital and Community Services Budget (%)	59.7	59.4

Source: House of Commons Health Committee, Memorandum from the Department of Health on Public Expenditure on Health & Social Services, Session 1993/94, HC617.

In the last few years, however, it has again become commonplace to talk in terms of a switch from acute to non-acute, or sometimes secondary to primary, or 'hospital to community' as though it were self-evidently correct. This general presumption contains a number of different elements which are often confused, even though they have very different policy implications:

- that better services outside hospital will reduce the need for hospital services;
- that some non-hospital services offer better value than hospital services;
- that some hospital services can be better provided in other settings.

In London, the Tomlinson Report (Department of Health, 1992), like previous reports into London's health services, suggested that one condition of reform of the hospital sector – in particular a reduction in its bed capacity – was a strengthening of general practice. The case for strengthening primary care in London rests mainly on its perceived low level of quality, but the report also argued that such improvements would reduce the workload of London's hospitals.

At the national level, there is no policy framework which sets out the need for such a switch in areas where GP services are already well organised. Indeed, at no time nor in any part of the country has the principle set out in the 1962 Plan – that hospitals should carry out only those functions which they were uniquely placed to discharge – been systematically implemented, nor has it been systematically evaluated. Rather, in some areas and for some services, individual clinicians or individual units have made their individual contribution to realising it by experimenting with new forms of services: at times the impetus has come from outside the hospital but in some areas hospitals themselves have introduced 'outreach' services. As for the diversion of resources away from hospitals because other uses are of greater value, again examples can be found where switches have been made, but the general pressure of Government policies in recent years has been in the direction of requiring hospitals to do more work so as to allow waiting lists and waiting times for elective surgery to be reduced. Against that background, switches of resources away from hospitals have been hard to achieve.

In the absence of any effective commitment to limiting the role of hospitals to what they alone can do, they have accumulated functions almost, it might be said, 'because they are there'. They were in the 1960s and they remain in the 1990s the largest health care delivery institutions and have therefore been the natural physical and organisational focus for service development. Within the old district structure, they were the dominant organisation, with community units often the poor relation. The latter were rarely, if ever, headed up by consultants. These spent virtually all their time within the confines of a hospital and effectively controlled the majority of the resources allocated to district health authorities. Against that background, it is not surprising that it was hard to effect changes in service patterns involving a switch of resources away from the hospital itself.

However, for a variety of reasons, the central position of the hospital is being challenged. The main immediate reason for the recent recognition lies with the 1990 reforms. Though not directed at service delivery patterns as such, they have radically altered the context in which all health providers work and created thereby the conditions within which change in the structure of provision can be realised. The separation of purchasers from providers has created a set of institutions in a position to weigh the value of different services and different modes of provision and to switch resources accordingly. Over the past three to four years, the belief that priority should be given to community and primary care services has become commonplace, both in government statements and statements of strategic intent on the part of purchasers.

Although a challenge is being mounted to the role of the hospital from other providers, there is also a need, created by technological, economic and other forces, to rethink the way that hospital services themselves are provided. In other words, whatever the role of other providers, hospitals will have to change. That is the message of a number of reports on hospital services which have appeared in recent years, but while they agree on that, they do not agree on what the new structure should be. In particular, as Table 1.9 shows, they come to different conclusions on the degree of concentration of activities on single sites and the division of functions between different types of facility. Some suggest the creation of units

Table 1.9: Hospital hierarchies: alternative views

	Catchment populations (millions)		
	Main	*Local*	*Other*
S E Thames	0.3(0.5)	?	Polyclinics Elective Units
Oxford	0.5-0.8	0.05	
NAHAT	2.0+	?	
Stapleton	2.25	0.2-0.3	

Source: South East Thames Regional Health Authority (1991), PN Dixon et al (1992), NAHAT (1993) and Templeton (1994)

serving very large catchment areas – up to two million people. Others propose 'main' hospitals, larger than the average DGH and smaller units specialising in different functions. More radically, Warner and Riley (1994) have suggested that the district general hospital should disappear, its functions split between local facilities and specialist centres: see Diagram 1.1.

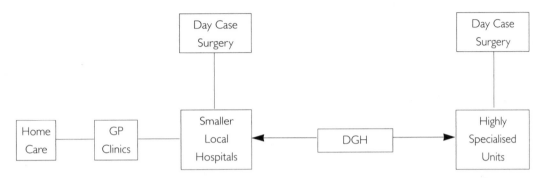

Diagram 1.1   The end of the district general hospital?

Other reports propose other, apparently different, forms of institution – intensive intervention centres, polyclinics, health maintenance centres, health villages, neighbourhoods or whatever. The very range reflects a general recognition that new patterns of service delivery are possible but at the same time considerable uncertainty as to what the best among the large range of possibilities should be. In addition, most of the main hospital specialties have put forward proposals for the way the services for which they are responsible should be structured; so have a number of reviews within London following Sir Bernard Tomlinson's report on London's hospitals. All agree that change is required.

Given the time that has elapsed since the last statement on hospital policy, this is hardly surprising. What is perhaps more surprising, given the scale of current investment in hospitals, is that there remains a policy vacuum at national level. Even though the 1962 Plan may well be regarded as an appropriate response to the conditions prevailing at the time, in the years since the Plan was formulated, the way hospitals function has been radically transformed. None of the specific assumptions made at that time, such as the number of beds needed to serve a particular population, remain valid as the technology of hospital care has transformed the way that hospital resources are used.

While technical and economic changes would in themselves compel a rethinking of the role of the hospital, another kind of pressure is equally important. It is now the conventional wisdom that the effectiveness of health care provision cannot be taken for granted; evidence on outcomes is required. The NHS Executive is now suggesting to purchasers (NHS Executive,

1994) that they base their decisions on what services to buy on such evidence; the NHS Research and Development Strategy is aimed at providing it. The authors of the 1962 Plan and subsequent revisions to it were of course looking for good outcomes but they lacked the means to demonstrate that what they proposed was better than some other configuration. Reliance on professional judgement was inevitable. In large measure that remains true, as the reports referred to in Table 1.1 indicate.

But while the terms of the debate are beginning to change, the essential structure has not. The 1962 Plan and subsequent modifications revolve around conflicting objectives of providing accessible services – which means small, local facilities – and good quality, which may mean large, district or regional facilities. At the same time, costs have got to be taken into account; good quality and good access may mean higher costs. But, while the tensions between cost, quality and access considerations remain, the context in which they operate has changed.

The immediate focus of hospital policy is not the same as in the 1960s. At that time, the central objective was to ensure a reasonable level of service in all parts of the country by ensuring that poorly served areas had a decent standard of facilities of their own. This required a large programme of new hospital building either on new sites or involving major rationalisation on existing sites. Now the emphasis is on reducing bed capacity in those areas, particularly the conurbations which, at least in terms of beds, are over-served and, particularly in London, on strengthening other parts of the health care system.

However, both then and now the same objectives can be identified: first, the hospital service should be of the right size relative to other forms of care and second, that hospital services should be structured in such a way as to offer the best chances of a high quality service within whatever level of resources is available. Clearly there are many determinants of the quality of hospital services – the skills of the medical and support staff, the abilities of managers and the equipment they have at their disposal and so on.

The concern of this report is much narrower. It focuses on two questions: is the notion of the district general hospital still valid and, if so, how should it relate to more specialised services on the one hand and to the services outside the hospital on the other? In attempting to answer these questions, we develop the basic framework, expressed in the 1962 Plan and other official reports through to the 1981 Consultation Document, which turns on getting the balance right between what may be the conflicting considerations of quality of care, cost of provision and access.

CHAPTER 2

Why general hospitals?

The case for providing care in the concentrated form known as a general hospital lies in the belief that links exist between the distinct functions which take place within it, which are important either because they lead to better quality of care or because they offer cost advantages. These links may be of various kinds – clinical, financial, managerial – and different considerations apply to each.

The activities which the general hospital links together are themselves diverse: they serve different markets, both in terms of scale and in terms of the nature of the needs they meet and in other ways too. Some activities are planned and can be precisely managed; others are inherently unpredictable. They use different technologies and different types of staff. Furthermore, the number of distinct activities which have to be accommodated within the same physical and managerial framework has been growing. Where once general hospitals were staffed by general physicians and surgeons covering a wide range of work, they now increasingly consist of groups of specialists in particular organs or client groups. Some 40 such groups now have official recognition in the UK as specialties.

Given this diversity, it is perhaps surprising that they fit together at all. The question, therefore, this chapter addresses is: what are the reasons for believing that this method of producing health care will produce advantages in terms of quality and cost? The framework it uses for thinking about this question is essentially the same as that underlying the official reports and other documents cited in Chapter 1. These assumed that hospitals of a certain size were essential to the provision of good quality care, but recognised that considerations of access and cost had also to be taken into account. This strategic trichotomy runs through all the documents cited in Chapter 1. But while it is central to the approach adopted in this report, it is pursued further by identifying trade-offs between these competing considerations below the level of the hospital itself, be it for particular specialties or groups of patients.

This chapter initially adopts, as did the 1962 Plan, a narrow definition of what is meant by clinical quality, focusing primarily on the treatment and procedures which hospitals provide and their outcomes, ignoring the other aspects of quality of care which users may consider important. This assumption is relaxed later on.

Cost is an omnipresent factor in any choice involving the use of resources, and needs no justification for its inclusion, but access deserves some elaboration. The need to consider access follows directly from our central focus on the structure of hospital provision. That concern is a spatial one: if there are 1,000 hospitals instead of 2,000, then inevitably the average distance that patients need to travel to a hospital will be higher. Whether this matters or not turns on the effect that distance – and its concomitant, cost of travel – has on the behaviour and the welfare of the potential hospital user and the extent to which any undesirable effects can be mitigated by suitable interventions to counter them.

At the same time, however, for patients needing care from more than one professional, the hospital may save on access costs by avoiding the need for trips to a number of different sites. The same is true for relationships between professionals within the hospital. Again, there are a number of distinct elements ranging from the effect of distance on staff recruitment and retention, to the physical advantages of having related activities on one site, to the less tangible advantages of clinicians and others having ready access to each other's expertise. Here, communication rather than physical proximity as such is what matters. In other words, the hospital can be seen as a device for reducing interaction costs between professionals.

This chapter explores the links between the three central elements – quality, cost and access – and the way that hospital services are configured, with the aim of identifying where they might run in conjunction and where they run in opposition. In the latter case, choices, or trade-offs between these three elements must be made.

2.1 What is a general hospital?

The central idea underlying the general, as opposed to the specialist, hospital is that there are benefits from providing a number of different services on the same site. These benefits were assumed in the 1962 Plan and in later documents to arise in two main ways: through better quality and lower costs. In other words, these two main elements of our analysis were assumed to run together, at least up to a point. The scope of the general hospital was defined by a range of specialties and support services, which it was judged every district should have; the scale was defined in terms of an appropriate medical staffing structure for those specialties. Scope, scale and other terms used in this chapter are briefly described in Box 2.1.

The general hospital by its nature is large in terms of scope, ie its range of activity comprises most medical specialties, as well as the support services these require. How large it must be in these terms to qualify as general is not a clear-cut matter. Curiously, given the central role the

> **Box 2.1 Terminology**
>
> ■ Scope refers to the range of specialties and other activities undertaken in a hospital. Economies of scope exist if costs fall or quality rises as the range widens.
>
> ■ Scale refers to the level of each activity- how many cases, how large the staff etc. Economies of scale exist if costs fall or quality rises as scale increases.
>
> ■ Clusters are groups of specialties and/or support activities: the larger a cluster the greater the scope of the hospital.
>
> ■ Concentration refers to bringing together staff and facilities associated with a particular specialty activity. Thus a single specialty hospital would be a concentrated form of provision if it was large relative to other providers of that specialty but the scope of such a hospital would be small.

concept of the DGH has played in British hospital planning, no formal definition appears to exist. Some of the terms used in the 1962 Plan and echoed in subsequent documents, such as general medicine and general surgery are fairly elastic in their meaning. Similarly, as noted earlier, the dividing line between general and specialist services is unclear.

One approach is to count as general a hospital which works in most of the areas of work defined for the purposes of recording clinical activity. Currently, the health resource group (HRG) is the most commonly used method: there are about 500 such groups (Sanderson *et al*, 1995). In 1991/92, there were a little over 200 hospitals in England carrying out work in 300 or more HRGs; taken together, they accounted for over 90 per cent of acute hospital activity. A few have merged since then, but the broad picture still holds.

At the other end of the scale, there are a large number of small hospitals working in a very narrow range of specialties. These hospitals are small in terms of scope and most are small in terms of scale, ie in the areas in which they work, they carry out only a modest number of operations or procedures relative to the general units. But some, the large single specialty hospitals, carry out similar amounts of work to the smaller general institutions. Within the 200 or so general units, differences in scope are fairly small, but there are considerable differences in scale. The largest carries out over 100,000 episodes per year; the smallest, about 10,000, depending on where the cut-off line distinguishing general from other hospitals is drawn. While the cut-off line may be hard to draw, any general hospital must be large in terms of scope, and so the chapter begins by identifying the links between size measured in these terms and the three central elements of the analysis – quality, cost and access. It then goes on to consider the largely different factors which determine the links between these and the scale of activity.

2.2 Scope

The assumption, implicit in the 1962 Plan and the 1980 Consultation Document, was that clinical quality would follow from the presence in a single (district) general hospital of most specialties, with a suitable staff structure for each together with the support services they required. In the words of the Plan:

> *The district general hospital offers the most practicable method of placing the full range of hospital services at the disposal of patients. (para 20)*

As the previous chapter indicated, that objective has now largely been achieved: a network of general hospitals supported by referral centres exists. The question now is whether the arguments underlying the 1962 approach remain valid. To answer it, we need to distinguish a number of different elements within the medical arguments for clustering specialties together and their relationship to the three central elements of our analysis: clinical quality, cost and access.

Clinical Quality

Perhaps the central argument for clustering is linked to the role of the hospital as a provider of emergency care. The essence of an emergency or accident is that the incident itself cannot be forecast and hence the appropriate response cannot be known in advance. Following this argument, the South East Thames analysis turns on the assumption that to cope with emergency admissions, a hospital must have available nearly the full range of medical expertise. As it puts it:

> *accident and emergency services need critically to be at single site hospitals with the following related acute specialties – general medicine, general surgery, paediatrics, trauma and orthopaedics, obstetrics and gynaecology, diagnostic and interventional radiology, anaesthetics, intensive care therapy, coronary care therapy. (SETRHA, 1991)*

Thus, the structure of the hospital is built up by considering what is needed to handle accident and emergency cases. Other specialties are then linked in because they have need of the same facilities, such as diagnostics and intensive care. The capacity to handle emergency cases on this view dominates the way that hospitals offering acute care should be configured.

However, the connections between the different parts of the hospital are not equally strong, nor are they of the same nature. All specialties may have a contribution to make to care for emergency cases – though to different degrees or for patients requiring treatment across specialties. In some cases, such as ENT, that contribution may be very rare; in others such as orthopaedics, it is central and hence appears in the South East Thames core list.

In other cases, particularly maternity and obstetrics, the links are primarily through the staff involved in both services. In yet other cases, the links are through the needs of the patient. For example, in the case of children, some forms of treatment, eg for childhood cancers, may provoke conditions which other specialties have to deal with. Such conditions are relatively rare. Most surgery on children, however, is performed by surgeons also operating on adults. But the aftercare or care in the event of an emergency developing is most appropriately offered by paediatricians. In this way, surgeons operating on children require a paediatric presence on site even though the converse may not be true.

At the other end of the age scale, similar issues may arise. *The Interface between Geriatric Medicine and General Medicine* (NHS Scotland, 1994) concluded:

15. The development of collaboration between geriatric medicine and general medicine has in the past been frustrated by logistic constraints. Historically, geriatric units have developed on sites separate from those of the related DGHs, making close co-operation between the specialties more difficult. This trend has however been reversed by the capital building programme for new DGHs, although separately-sited units still operate in some, mainly teaching hospitals.

16. The advantages of same site developments are:

- *closer contact, formal and informal, between geriatricians and other specialists, leading to ease of referral and transfer across specialties, and early assessment of patient's total care needs*
- *access to a comprehensive range of on-site investigative facilities*
- *availability of day care and outpatient facilities for the elderly acute patient*
- *integration of junior staff rotas in the specialties of geriatric and general medicine, particularly to allow cross cover.*

Similar statements on the linkages between different hospital functions can be found in the London speciality reviews (London Implementation Group 1993 a–f). Taken together they suggest that, by one route or another, all hospital specialties and facilities are inter-linked either directly or indirectly through use of common facilities or specialties such as anaesthesia on which they rely.

These arguments do not apply to the third main type of medical work, consultation and diagnosis, at least not in most cases. The clinical case for physical proximity turns on the availability of the doctor providing consultation and diagnostic services for inter-professional consultation or, in the event of an emergency elsewhere in the hospital, medical cover as well.

Most emergency admissions are medical cases: the majority of surgical procedures are carried out on an elective or planned basis. However, here too unpredictability is pertinent but in a different sense. While the nature of the intervention required is known in advance, the condition of the patient may not be: there is always the risk that 'something may go wrong' and hence that the full emergency resources such as intensive care units and specialist medical and nursing skills may be required to rectify it. A study of intensive care beds (McKee and Black 1995) found that out of 200 patients included in a census of one day's activity, 24 were admitted as emergency care after elective surgery and a further 61 were elective or expected admissions after elective surgery.

The case for clustering in respect of planned work thus has two components: the difficulty of predicting in advance what may happen and the risks of dealing with an emergency situation in an institution not appropriately equipped for this purpose. Transfer between hospitals is always possible and in some cases will be perfectly feasible and effectively risk-free. In others, the delay and other consequences may be critical, and hence physical proximity is vital.

But exactly what is meant by proximity, and how important it is, is hard to pin down precisely as the following example illustrates. In their discussion of the handling of major injuries, the British Orthopaedic Association and the British Association of Plastic Surgeons (1993) emphasise the need for close links between orthopaedic and plastic surgeons, proposing that a joint treatment plan should be drawn up between plastic and orthopaedic surgeons.

As the extract in Box 2.2 indicates, physical proximity is advantageous, making consultation easier and reducing the time lost in achieving it. But a joint treatment plan can nevertheless be drawn up without it. In other circumstances, however, physical separation may be critical. We noted earlier that in the 1980s, the district general hospital was turned into an organisational concept rather than a physical one, so services were, or remained, divided over more than one site. The result, criticised for the risks it created for emergency care, was that medical cover was also split and as a result, decisions on how to treat patients were made by junior doctors not experienced enough to do so well. As a result, the quality of care provided was well below what hospitals elsewhere could provide.

Box 2.2 Treatment plans

- The purpose of the communication is the joint production of a treatment plan for the first 5 days. Thus the minimum response from the plastic surgery service is advice. Ideally the plastic surgeon, like the orthopaedic consultant, should have an interest in severe lower limb injuries. Where the two specialties are on the same site it should be possible for them to examine the patient together shortly after admission. It is more difficult when the specialties are on split sites. This, however, is no reason or excuse for there not being a joint approach to the management.

- A telephone discussion may be all that is necessary to formulate a joint plan. If the surgeons involved are used to managing trauma cases together, a telephone discussion will establish the likely tissue defect, the likely bone fixation and the likely type of plastic reconstruction required. Where there is any doubt about the requirements of the plastic surgery, then there is no alternative but for the plastic surgeon to see the patient before or in the early stages of the first operation. This may pose considerable problems to the plastic surgeon because of travelling and the interruption of other work, but the benefits of embarking on a well thought out line of treatment are so great that it should be given the highest priority (p 3).

Source: British Orthopaedic Association and British Association of Plastic Surgeons (1993)

Similarly, the case for providing 24-hour consultant cover for emergency care rests on the belief that the highest level of expertise must be immediately available, not on call at home or in a nearby hospital. The justification for that remains to be demonstrated, but these examples are sufficient to show that proximity requires careful analysis to determine what precisely it means, when it is important and when not.

Finally, the hospital is an institution for the dissemination and creation of knowledge as well as its application. Hence there should be benefits in having different specialties interacting with each other informally, or formally through medical audit. The argument here turns on the nature of the hospital as an institution for the creation and exchange of knowledge and encouragement to innovation. The boundaries between specialties are fluid and the needs of many patients run across them. Clustering promotes, though it does not guarantee, cross-fertilisation of ideas and hence the quality of care. This way of putting the argument, it is worth noting, implicitly values the links between hospital professions highly while, at best, being neutral about the importance of other professional links, ie with those working in other locations.

While dissemination between experienced professionals is important to the maintenance of their clinical skills, the general hospital can also be seen as a device for collecting the human wherewithal for the teaching of medical students, allowing as it does immediate and convenient access to a wide range of conditions requiring diagnosis and treatment. In the 19th century, the development of specialist hospitals was regarded with hostility by the majority of doctors working in general hospitals in part for this very reason. In more recent times, the viability of particular hospital configurations may depend on the the mix of patients they can provide for teaching purposes. Whether this link between care and teaching requirements is inherent or artificial is considered in Chapter 9.

So far we have considered medical staff. But support staff, diagnostic and other specialist facilities must be physically close so that when the unexpected arises and has to be dealt with immediately, or the need to consult colleagues occurs, both can be done promptly. Physically close is of course not a precise term: in the case of staff, it may mean face to face or it may mean 'on call at home' or even at another nearby hospital. In some cases, the sample taken from a patient for testing must be literally 'hot' and analysed very close to the patient. In others, there is time for results to be obtained from a physically distant site. Similarly, patients may be transferred to where the necessary facilities for diagnostic or intensive care exist. But that takes time and may also involve risks to the patient. Indeed, according to the British Paediatric Association (1993), such risks may occur within hospitals because:

> *Children's wards may be located at some distance from other departments in the hospital, and, in the event of an acute emergency, immediate availability of anaesthetic and other appropriate help cannot always be guaranteed. (p 6)*

The same study also found that:

> *For well over half of the instances in which critically ill children were transferred from one hospital to another, this was accomplished by a locally organised ad hoc team from the referring hospital, commonly with inadequate staff numbers, training, resources and equipment. (p 9)*

But proximity is not solely a geographical concept. Modern communications technologies can convey cheaply and rapidly the results of x-rays or other diagnostics from where they are taken to where they can be interpreted. As a result, in some circumstances distance is immaterial, even if it remains critical in others. As the London Specialty Review Group for Neurosciences put it:

Expert radiological opinion can be obtained from the tertiary centre and current developments in wide area networking enable imaging and other electronic data to be relayed from the district general hospital direct to the centre, thereby providing rapid access to specialist opinion. (para 63)

As a result, the need for close physical proximity is removed.

Costs

The central cost argument for clustering turns on the advantages in terms of shared facilities in producing what may or may not be related services on one site. For example, all specialties may share a pathology laboratory or diagnostic equipment, even if patients are not transferred between them. Their co-existence may create enough demand to justify the use of expensive and high-capacity equipment or other overhead costs. In this way, the clinical scope of a hospital creates a scale economy in a support service.

Second, proximity may mean that services are cheaper to provide because transport costs are avoided. This may be true of catering services although recent development such as freezing and packaged meals have tended to work the other way. Thus, there can be no general expectation that on-site is cheaper. There is nothing in the nature of the hospital as such which determines whether, for example, food should be prepared inside it or brought to it. Rather the question turns on the technology of that particular service: whether it allows off-site provision and whether it is subject to economies of scale at levels of provision greater than the individual hospital itself requires.

A further argument links costs with more general considerations about how hospitals should be organised; it depends not so much on proximity as on the nature of the links between different services. In the 1980s, the idea of general management has been implemented precisely in order to strengthen the connections between the different functions of the hospital. Put (over)simply, the Government took the view that unless there was an identifiable chain of command, it would not be possible to raise the level of hospital efficiency. However, another Government initiative, competitive tendering for support services, pushed the other way, by introducing the idea that activities within the hospital could be integrated by contract rather than by a single line of management. The NHS and Community Care Act 1990 has led in a few areas to clinical work being put out to tender as well.

The relative merits of these two forms of structure require assessment on a case by case basis.

Robinson (1994) has argued that where links between functions are close but not always easy to predict, and hence subject to variation, eg most work connected with emergencies, integrated management within a single organisation may be more effective than co-ordinating separate supplying units through contracts. However, it remains an open question whether or not integrated management itself requires physical integration into one institution. As noted already, many hospital trusts operate on several sites: whether they would perform better in managerial terms if they were clustered on one site is hard to judge on a general basis. Furthermore, the force of this argument turns critically on the nature of the links involved, in particular, for some services links between hospitals may be as important as links within them, a point considered further below.

Fourth, where users must make use of a range of services at more or less the same time, it may be convenient in terms of access to visit them on one site, ie it may reduce the number of trips the user must make. For example, the diabetic patient may need to see a physician but also a podiatrist. Thus clustering may reduce as well as increase access costs for some users.

To conclude the discussion of scope: clusters can be justified in a number of different ways: the need to cluster is not the same for all the services which a hospital comprises or at all times or for all patients. A general way of expressing the case for clustering is in terms of risk: the larger the cluster, the greater the chances that the relevant skills and services will be available for whatever conditions a patient presents and the lower the chances of transfer to other facilities being required. The other side of the coin is that for many patients and services, only a small part of what the hospital can provide is required and their needs can be forecast accurately in advance by their referring GP or, indeed, in the case of chronic patients familiar with their own conditions, themselves. Thus, outpatient consultations do not contribute to clinical advantages of scope except insofar as the physical presence of a consultant may be important for inter-professional consultation. But any specialty or support service which may, even if rarely, contribute to emergency care, does.

2.3 Scale

So far we have aimed to distinguish the range or scope of activity from the scale at which each is carried out. In the 1962 Plan, the distinction was ignored: the scale of the hospital emerged from a consideration of the range of activity to be included in it, and then scale was determined by considering how each activity should be staffed and how much work each staff team could do. In effect this amounted to treating the staff team as a fixed cost, to be spread over a reasonable workload, but it also contained the judgement that once a hospital had reached a satisfactory scope and was staffed accordingly, there was no case for going bigger. Thus, the district general hospital defined in the 1962 Plan was the smallest compatible with its broad objective of providing each district with the broad range of hospital services. But that left out the possibility that quality might be increased and cost reduced by hospitals that were much larger than the minimum. On both grounds, therefore, scale must be considered in its own right.

Clinical Quality

The approach in the 1962 Plan was, in essence, to assume that if each specialty was staffed properly, good quality care would follow. The same approach also lies behind the other planning documents cited in the previous chapter. In the case of the South East Thames Strategy, the scale of the emergency hospital depends directly on the volume of resources required to provide an adequate accident and emergency facility. In particular, the report suggests that if it turns out that trauma centres perform well, then the maximum size of the hospital should be increased. The advantages of these turn in part on having the range of skills on one site, ie the scope of the hospital, but also on its scale. The larger the hospital in terms of its medical staffing, the easier it is to ensure that those skills are available at all times, simply because cross-cover is easier to arrange.

However, the link between scale and quality may work in other ways. In recent years, analysts of actual hospital performance have approached the issue by comparing the results of what hospitals do with various characteristics of the hospital, including its size and volume of work. That work, reviewed in more detail in Chapter 5, suggests that there is a relationship, though not always a strong one, between the volume of activity, usually the number of patients in a particular category treated, and the quality, usually measured by mortality rates, of the work done.

The hypothesis that scale of activity and quality of outcome are linked is often termed 'practice makes perfect', reflecting the common sense view that if people do more of a particular procedure, they get better at doing it. This form of scale benefit may not only apply to the individual surgeon or physician but also to the wider team including nursing and administrative support on which they rely.

However, scale and quality may be linked in other ways too. Put simply, the larger the hospital in terms of patients treated, the greater the scope for specialisation among its medical and its support staff. Similarly, the larger the catchment, the greater the chances of its staff seeing rare conditions with sufficient frequency to be able to diagnose and treat them effectively. If specialisation is critical to quality, then the larger the population catchments and the larger the hospitals have to be in order to allow specialisation to take place – assuming for the moment that all services have to be within one institution. The authors of the 1962 Plan recognised at that time that the growth of medical knowledge was in turn leading to a growth in specialisms. That process has continued, leading to sub-division in existing specialties and the virtual elimination of the general physician or surgeon, at least in larger institutions. This process can be described as extending the scope of the hospital by extending the range of specialties it comprises or enlarging the scale of each specialty. Either way, the effect is to increase the minimum size of the hospital at which all specialties are represented.

The second key element is the size of each team: how large does a group within a specialty have to be? In part, this merges into the previous question, ie it becomes a question of definition of 'sub-specialty'. Take ophthalmology – a small specialty in terms of consultant numbers – which comprises work of a number of distinct kinds. A recent statement by the Royal College of Ophthalmologists (1993) identifies the need for specialists in particular procedures – eight areas in all. This degree of specialisation, which the College believes necessary for a good quality service, can only be achieved in hospitals with large catchment areas.

> *There will always be patients requiring the skill of an ophthalmologist specialising in a particular aspect of the subject such as complex corneal surgery, neuro-opthalmology, medical ophthalmology, vitreo-retinal surgery, orbital surgery and difficult ocular motility problems. This specialist care will be required in large urban communities where it can best be provided by eye hospitals or large ophthalmic departments within general hospitals. These hospitals or departments inevitably need a higher level of both trained staff and of staff in training, in order that these special activities can be taught and developed. They also require, in those specialties that are surgically orientated, additional operating facilities. Patients with these complicated conditions also require much more intensive investigation and their care and treatment is much more time consuming (p 9).*

How large is large? Suffice to say here, that although the case for larger teams and greater specialisation runs through most specialty reviews, their views on optimal population catchment areas do not coincide, nor is there any reason to expect they should. Different specialties serve very different populations and draw on distinct bodies of knowledge and technique.

Cost

There may be economies of scale in any of the services the hospital requires: its heating plant, its laundry equipment, and so on. In these cases economies may arise not so much through fixed costs being spread over more output, but because of the nature of the technologies concerned. In general, the efficiency of heating plants increases with size so cost per unit of heating falls as the amount supplied increases. In other cases, economies may result through spreading the cost of certain fixed assets such as diagnostic equipment which requires high utilisation levels if it to be justified. In this and other cases, the issue is purely an empirical one.

The same type of argument applies to workforce costs. If, to provide a satisfactory service, a minimum number of staff are required, a threshold or critical mass is created, below which it will be either inefficient to work or quality is likely to be poor. The general argument may apply to any aspect of the hospital, but as far as quality of care is concerned, the critical threshold is that relating to emergency care. The essence of a hospital providing emergency care is that it is a 24-hour, 365-day facility: the level of this threshold depends critically on the range of specialties required and level at which each can provide cover of whatever is the appropriate standard. The greater the emphasis on the need to provide highly skilled staff – ie consultant level or equivalent – at all times, the larger the complement required within each speciality and hence the larger the threshold at which a high quality service can be provided.

Although this is the central argument relating to size, economies of scale in the hospital can arise in other ways. First, learning by doing may apply to cost as well as quality. The more of a particular activity a hospital takes on, the lower its costs should be by virtue of the staff – medical, nursing and technical – becoming more skilled at it. Furthermore, the greater the scale, the greater the degree of specialisation that is feasible and hence of learning by doing.

Second, a large unit can deal better with variability in demand than a small one. The larger the unit, the cheaper it is to ensure a given level of availability. This is not just a matter of how much physical capacity must be available, but also of staffing levels. Although idle time can be cut by appropriate staffing policies, such as use of part-time staff, there are limits to what can be done to reduce it while still maintaining adequate cover, particularly medical and other specialised staff. Hence larger units will be more economic.

The number of beds required to guarantee a given risk rises less than proportionately to the numbers served as pointed out in *Emergency Pathways* (King's Fund, 1994), a study of accident and emergency care in London:

> *The overall number of beds which need to be provided to cope with unpredictable acute admissions declines with the size of the admitting unit. For example, the mean number of expected emergency admissions in an area of London in one year might be 36,500 patients; in any 24-hour period this would suggest that 100 patients will need beds. However, this latter figure is a 'sample' drawn from the year total and will have confidence intervals associated with it. Thus, for a mean expected figure of 100 patients, there might be a 95 per cent chance that the actual figure will be between 95 and 105 in any 24-hour period. In other words, for this level of 'safety' there would have to be 105 beds provided to cope with all but one in twenty situations.*

> *An individual hospital might expect some 20 of these overall expected 100 patients to be referred to it: but this 'sample' would carry relatively high confidence intervals of, say, 10 to 30 to contain 95 per cent of likely admissions. For an individual ward the mean might be only 5 patients but with confidence intervals of between 0 and over 20. Thus, whereas an area of London would need to provide 105 beds, if care were provided by entirely separate hospitals, there would have to be 150 beds available in total, and if by individuals wards, some 400 or so. In other words, the overall resources needed to cope with the unpredictability of acute emergency admissions decreases significantly the larger the admitting unit. (p 29.*

This source of scale advantage does not apply to all hospital activities. It is important for a range of services, including for example intensive care facilities and accident and emergency care, but largely irrelevant to elective activities and consultations since these can be managed on a planned basis which allows utilisation to be geared to the capacity available.

Another utilisation argument turns not on risk and uncertainty but on the optimal use of a professional's time. Many services currently based in hospitals involve professionals giving advice and providing simple treatment. The argument for these activities taking place in a general hospital is that this is the best way of using professional time: time spent travelling between patients is eliminated. In this way, the hospital is a device for saving professional time at the expense of users who have to meet the costs of access. Many services like physiotherapy or routine consultations can be provided off-site or at home. But in hospital cost terms, it may be less expensive to keep them in-house. This point has been cogently put by the Association of Dermatologists (undated) in the following terms:

> *The British Association of Dermatologists feels strongly that in the vast majority of cases the*

pressure on its members to perform community clinics is inappropriate and not to the medium or long term advantage of the patients themselves. The status of British dermatology is high because, over the past twenty years or more, consultants have moved away from being peripatetic specialists, without a firm base, who travelled from hospital to hospital to being integrated members of a hospital team where they can teach, carry out research and audit and play a full part in the planning and management of healthcare provision. The introduction of community clinics is therefore seen as a retrograde step, weakening the specialty.

On the other hand, the *Report of the Review of London Renal Services* (London Implementation Group, 1993f) argued:

Renal medicine is a complex specialty and a concentration of activities is necessary to provide sufficient consultant staff for continuous cover, and for the support and training of both junior doctors and other professional staff. Increasing sub-specialisation also points to the need for a tertiary centre to be staffed by a number of consultants. A corollary of such a concentration of staff is the requirement that they provide outreach services (support for satellite dialysis units, and out-patient clinics) so as to permit the ready access of patients to the facilities they require. (para 5)

As these quotations show, there are conflicts between cost and quality on the one hand and access on the other. To ensure the latter, the professionals' time may have to be 'wasted' through lower levels of utilisation. These trade-offs are explored further below.

To sum up the discussion of scale: as with scope, there are different strands to the scale argument which impact on different services in different ways. In particular, some suggest there will be cost thresholds below which services are likely to be expensive to provide, particularly where expensive equipment is concerned or where clinical teams must be of a certain size to ensure the presence of the appropriate skills at all relevant times. Above those thresholds, scale benefits may continue to accrue but there is no reason why advantages of scale, where they exist, should coincide for each of the vast range of services that a hospital provides. The optimal grouping for any one specialty turns on the range of expertise *it* comprises and the scale of the demand for *its* services.

If hospital services must be clustered, then the scale of the hospital as a whole is determined by the scale of the smaller specialties such as neurosurgery, where catchment populations are measured in millions. Put more broadly, the development of interdependence between specialties and the growth of specialties combine to create a case for larger and larger institutions as they undermine the generalist's role in providing emergency medical and surgical cover for a wide range of eventualities. But there are arguments working the other way and it is these which we turn to next.

2.4 Limits to scope and scale

If quality increases with scope and size, and costs fall or remain constant, then there is, in McKeown's words (1965), no upper limit to the size of the hospital. As far as costs are concerned, the Bonham-Carter Report (DHSS, 1969) for example assumed that the concentration implied by the district general hospital would reduce them. Later documents took a more sceptical view, suggesting that costs might start to rise as scale increased. The arguments suggesting an upper limit to size fall into two categories: diseconomies either of scope or scale within the hospital and the costs of access to the hospital, primarily for patients but also for staff.

Diseconomies of scope and scale

The modern hospital is a large and complex institution. It is one which experience has shown is hard to manage, not simply by virtue of its scale and diversity but also because of the competing professional and managerial hierarchies it embodies. On this view it would seem a reasonable assumption that unit costs might grow with size because the larger the institution, the harder it is to manage, particularly if extension of scope goes hand in hand with scale. The Royal Commission (DHSS, 1979) suggested that 'The larger the DGH... the more serious the problems of communication within it.' The 1980 Consultation Document rephrased essentially the same point by suggesting that over a certain point extra costs arise within the hospital, which becomes more and more difficult to manage as size increases.

> *Experience has shown that a large degree of concentration on a single site may itself have serious disadvantages. Communications of all kinds within the hospital become more complex and difficult, as does management. Patients and relatives, as well as staff, find the hospital too impersonal. It often suffers from physical disadvantages such as distance between different departments and the need to provide air conditioning to internal areas, with high energy requirements. It is sometimes supposed that one building is cheaper to build and run than two, of equivalent functional content, but this may not always be the case. (para 10)*

No specific evidence was given to justify the arguments in this paragraph but it apparently reflects the judgement of many closely involved with the large units that emerged in the early 1970s.

The Consultation Document used these arguments to justify retention of smaller general hospitals to support the main unit in a district. But equally, it could be used to justify a different kind of separation, such as one based on a functional split eg between emergency and elective work, provided that the units so created were 'manageable'.

Hughes and Allen (1993) suggest that because of their complexity, hospital services might be disaggregated in order to ease the problems of internal governance.

> *There appears to be significant scope in the UK for a disaggregation of hospital services so that certain specialties move out with the larger organisation to become self-contained, community facilities. In the USA this trend has had some negative consequences because it has often been motivated by the wish to move payments out from under the DRG system. However, free-standing units appear to have advantages both in terms of cost and ease of governance. Existing British day surgery units have proved to be an extremely cost-effective alternative to in-patient care. A growth of out-of-hospital care on the North American model might sidestep many of the problems that we have highlighted. (p 28)*

On the other hand, the South East Thames Strategy cites the two largest (in terms of beds) English hospitals, St James' Leeds and Queen's Medical Centre Nottingham, and suggests that there is no evidence that their performance has suffered from their size. However, while that may be true, the scale of some hospitals does undermine some of the advantages that might be claimed for clustering. Above a certain point, impossible to define numerically, the informal interactions essential to the collegiate role of the hospital that clustering may promote are likely to decline.

Arguments of this kind are inherently difficult to pin down precisely. Hospitals, like firms or government departments, may be structured in a variety of different ways to achieve what is judged to be the best balance between central control and greater freedom for decision making 'down the line'. For example, a division between emergency and planned work could be achieved by physical division, or by managerial separation within the same physical environment: it is impossible to show *a priori* which is superior.

It is not just links within the hospital, however, that may be affected by size. For many patients, particularly the seriously ill or the frail elderly, links between hospital and other services are central to the quality of care they receive. It is at least arguable that the larger the hospital, the harder those links will be to maintain, at least within the current conventions as to how hospitals should be organised, which emphasise the importance of internal relationships.

Formal management and communication systems can of course work to overcome any such tendency. But many of the contacts between hospital based doctors and others, including general practitioners and community nursing staff, work by virtue of informal contact and mutual trust. Both are arguably more likely to arise in smaller institutions.

Access Costs

While the existence of an upper limit set by management considerations may be controversial and hard to identify, it is self-evident and unavoidable that greater concentration of activity imposes access costs. The greater the concentration of facilities, the smaller the number of hospitals, the further people have to travel, including both workers, patients and those visiting them. Their travel costs, or those falling on the hospital, will therefore be higher.

So much is obvious. Nevertheless, the nature of the link between concentration and access costs needs some disentangling, since while it is clear that concentration will tend to raise access costs, it does so in different ways, and different kinds of evidence are relevant to determining the importance of each. Three kinds of cost need to be distinguished.

- *Costs to the NHS*: these include provision of ambulances, car services and payment of travel expenses. Clearly the greater the catchment area for a hospital, the greater these will be.
- *Costs of travel to patients and friends*: the costs of travel in terms of money, time and general inconvenience which must be met by patients and their visitors; these too will rise with catchment area.
- *Clinical Costs*: for emergencies such as road accident victims, the time taken to reach an accident and emergency facility may be critical to survival. The fewer the number of hospitals, the longer it would seem these trips would be. The issue, however, is not a straightforward matter of how long it takes for an ambulance to respond to an emergency call and make the trip to hospital. The essence of an emergency is that the need for treatment cannot be known accurately in advance. Unless all hospitals have the same facilities, then a serious accident raises the question, which the ambulance staff must solve, of which hospital the patient should be taken to. Travel to the nearest hospital may, in these circumstances, mean that transfer is required to one which is more suitably equipped. Overall journey time may in fact be increased at least for those patients where the question 'which hospital' is not easy even for trained staff to answer.

Longer access times and longer journeys may impose costs in other ways. For some patients, such as those requiring renal dialysis, the experience of that combined with a long trip at either end of the day may negate the value of the treatment. For children, the issue may be the 'costs' of separation from parents. The official recommendations for the care of children in hospital has been for 30 years, since publication of the Platt report (Ministry of Health 1959) been based on the view that such costs are high. Distance and difficulty of travel makes it hard for parents to keep in regular contact with their children (prior to the Platt report, it was common practice for parents to be discouraged from visiting). Overnight beds are now often provided to make it easier, thus replacing one type of cost with another. As the British Paediatric Association puts it (personal communication, 1994):

> *When children, necessarily, are admitted to hospital it is essential there is ease of access for their families, for the carer to be resident and support them during the care period and for the parent or carer to maintain close links with their own family home. Thus accessibility becomes a critical factor.*

Finally, clinical costs may arise if people are deterred from being treated by the costs and time involved in gaining access to hospital facilities. Transport planners invariably find that distance does deter travel. They also find, however, that its impact depends on the purpose for which trips are made: commuting trips are less sensitive to distance than shopping trips. If, as we might expect, trips to hospitals come at the less sensitive end of the spectrum, then distance will not impose great clinical costs. However, transport planners also find, not unexpectedly, that sensitivity to distance depends on income. On this basis, the clinical costs of distance are likely to be greater for lower income groups.

The first two categories of access cost are essentially of the same kind – the difference lies in who provides and pays for the transport facilities required. The third is different: it suggests that access difficulties may increase the clinical risks to patients or reduce the level of service they enjoy. Those costs are likely to be highest for accident victims or other emergency cases where the time between accident and treatment may be vital or for the sick and physically frail for whom the journey itself may be a trial, and for those on low incomes who find it hard to pay bus or taxi fares.

If as a result some do not use services as much as their needs suggest they should, then there are risks of poorer health for the individuals concerned. More generally, a fundamental objective of the NHS, equal access for equal need, will be undermined. It also means that the clinical advantages of clustering must be set against the access disadvantage it creates.

2.5 Conclusion

The main conclusion to emerge from this chapter is that the strands which bind the activities of the general hospital together are of different kinds and of varying importance. In some cases, clinical considerations may be decisive, in others costs, and in yet others the requirements of teaching and research. In some cases, such as emergency care, the linkages are strong; in others, such as diagnosis and consultation, relatively weak.

Clustering activities together imposes access costs, of either a monetary or a clinical kind, so trade-offs have to be made between the benefits of clustering and the benefits of access. Trade-offs between quality and costs of service provision may also arise. As the benefits of clustering vary between different hospital functions, it follows that the trade-offs between quality and access will vary from function to function. Thus, the general hospital represents a set of compromises between different considerations, both overall and for particular services or patient groups.

The question we turn to next is whether the single general hospital represents the best compromise. If different hospital functions have different characteristics, then the creation of separate clusters carrying out separate functions may allow a better balance between quality, cost and access to be struck for each of them. Put simply, if the clustering benefits are slight but the costs of access high, then the case for that particular function being included in the ambit of the general hospital is relatively weak. How different clusters can be justified is the subject of the next chapter.

CHAPTER 3

Systems of hospitals

There is clearly no reason why the three main functions of the acute hospital – emergency care, elective surgery and outpatient consultations – should have similar economic and clinical characteristics. All they do have in common, within the British hospital system, is that they are normally carried out by the same people working within the same institution.

As the modern hospital comprises a vast range of different services within each of these three main groups, it would be highly improbable that the optimum point, defined either as minimum cost or highest clinical quality or as some balance between accessibility and the other two objectives, would coincide at one particular level for all of them. Different specialties draw on different, if related, bodies of knowledge and they serve different groups of patients, some treating very common conditions, other less common and some very rare ones.

Within the framework set out in Chapter 2, the division of functions into distinct clusters can be seen as the obvious response to differences in the economic and clinical characteristics of different elements of hospital work. If each specialty had its own optimal balance between cost, quality and access, then what is best for each might be a single specialty hospital like those for eye care, cancer care and orthopaedics and ENT which still exist in some parts of the country.

On the other hand, if the clustering and concentration arguments were taken as decisive, then the outcome would be a single very large hospital. Whether that would lead to higher costs of provision is an open question, but it would certainly impose high access costs on patients. No such hospital exists in the UK, but some services such as neurosciences are provided only at the regional level; if it were vital that these should always co-exist with other specialties, then the result would be a small number of very large hospitals serving catchment areas of two or more million people.

The system of hospital provision that currently exists represents a compromise between these two extremes. The district general hospital clusters together most hospital functions, but others are only to be found on a smaller number of sites. This arrangement, usually termed a hierarchy, underlies the 1962 Hospital Plan and most official policy statements since. As Fox

(1986) has shown, the concept of a hierarchy has underpinned thinking about hospital policy for most of this century, both within the UK and the US. But for the most part, the concept has largely gone unexamined. While the need for a compromise between the competing considerations of quality and access is obvious enough, the different proposals set out in Table 1.9 above indicate that, within the same general approach, quite different hospital systems can be proposed. Furthermore, although all four sets of proposals listed embody the notion of a hierarchy, divisions on other grounds are also proposed, such as centres specialising in elective work or diagnostics, ie clusters based on a broadly defined function.

How hospital activities should be divided up is considered in the first part of this chapter. Once different hospitals perform different functions, then two further questions arise: how do patients find their way to the 'right' hospital and how do hospitals providing different but complementary services relate to each other? These are considered in the second part of the chapter.

3.1 Division of functions

The acute general hospital is based on the assumed advantages of clustering – scope – and concentration – scale. The case for providing some functions in other locations rests on two different sets of arguments:

- these advantages are not important for some functions and hence they can be carried out elsewhere – we term these separable functions;
- the DGH is not large enough for some functions to enjoy fully the advantages that large scope and high concentration can bring – we term these more specialised functions.

We take these in turn.

Separable Functions

The Oxford Strategy defines a range of services which can be provided away from the DGH: see Table 3.1. These include parts of longer care episodes such as diagnosis before admission and care after admission and the simpler parts of functions the bulk of which remain in the DGH: casualty, low risk maternity, and (simple) elective surgery.

For functions in the first group, separability is defined by analysing the process of care and

Table 3.1   Local services: Oxford strategy

Casualty

Short stay nursing beds

Radiology facilities

Basic pathology

Outpatient assessment and consultation

Elective surgery

Low risk recovery beds

Physiotherapy, occupational therapy, speech therapy and chiropody

Low risk maternity

Other primary and community facilities

Source: PN Dixon et al (1992)

identifying those elements where neither clustering nor scale arguments are significant. The effectiveness of a test depends largely on the skills of those executing it and the performance of the relevant equipment. Similarly, the bulk of consultations can be performed as well offsite as onsite. Only in a few cases are the special facilities of the hospital itself required.

For the second group the question of whether they are separable turns on the likelihood of risks to life or health occurring. For the bulk of hospital medical functions, whether there is or not scope for separation is not a clear-cut matter but one of degree of acceptable risk. Maternity services illustrate the difficulties in drawing a clear line very sharply. The model that developed over the past 30 or so years which involved centralising virtually all births in hospitals under the control of consultant obstetricians has been based on the view that everything should be done to eliminate risk. In the words of a spokesperson for the Royal College of Gynaecologists before the House of Commons Health Select Committee (1992):

> *It would seem to us clear that we feel that the safest place is where the facilities are. The finest of facilities will be in the biggest units. Fairly good facilities will be in much smaller units, but those facilities will be better, we believe, than no facilities at home, other than a flying squad and support of that kind. (p 392)*

The counterview is that in most cases risks are low and generally forecastable. Hence separation of care for some patients into a home or other 'low tech' environment can be achieved. Whether they are may be hard to resolve. In contrast to the views of the Royal College, the National Perinatal Epidemiology Unit (1994) argued that:

There is no evidence to support the claim that the safest policy is for all women to give birth in hospital. (p 119)

But even if the risks of giving birth outside a hospital are higher, some women may be willing to run them. Thus in this case, whether the service is in part separable turns on defining what the risks are and then allowing women to choose in the light of them.

In the case of elective work, the scope for separability turns on the ability of clinicians to define a range of procedures which reduces the risk of the basic back-up resources of the hospital being required to a negligible level and allows them to be confident that, if mishaps occur, those resources can be reached by transferring the patient safely to them. At the extreme, there is no doubt that can be done for very simple procedures such as those carried out in GPs' surgeries. But how far along the continuum towards complexity it is feasible to go is not clear cut, in part because of differences in clinical view as to what is 'complex' and risky, in part because, as with maternity care, some patients may be prepared to trade risk off against other advantages.

In the South East Thames Strategy, it was proposed that the line should be drawn through agreement of treatment protocols which would define on a case-by-case basis where the appropriate place of treatment would be. In the Oxford Strategy, it was assumed that the line should be drawn by the individual consultant who would decide whether to treat a patient in a general hospital with most support facilities to hand or in a local hospital with fewer. In neither case, however, was evidence put forward to show exactly what the risks were.

There is scope for separation within emergency work as well. A number of hospitals provide emergency services for a limited number of hours a day and covering only a limited range of conditions. For minor injuries – the walking wounded – it may be left to the patients, as it is for nurse-run casualty clinics, to allocate themselves appropriately. For more serious cases, how successful such specialisation is depends on the skills of the ambulance crews and their ability to determine to which hospital a patient should be directed or on the extent to which they can be controlled centrally and advised by radio or other means.

Up to this point the potential for separating out some general hospital functions has been examined by looking at simpler activities or parts of those which form parts of complex episodes of care. In the case of mental health services, opinion has been moving in favour of separation for the speciality as a whole. In the 1960s, the inclusion of mental illness beds within the district general hospital was seen as a means of raising the quality of care for this group of patients. It was also justified by the importance for some patients, such as those suffering from self-inflicted wounds or drug overdoses, of ready access to emergency facilities. Thus, in the words of the Review of Scotland's Hospital Plan (Scottish Home and Health Department, 1966):

> *Virtually all of the new general hospital will contain acute psychiatric units and this will greatly facilitate co-operation between psychiatry and other specialities. (para 26)*

In the last 30 years, attitudes and policy objectives have changed in favour of community-based provision: the advantages of integration with the rest of the acute hospital are less apparent and the risks to patients – because of the nature of the design of some acute hospitals – of that integration more apparent. The separate institution appears to offer an environment which is more conducive for patients to make the transition when on 'day release' to 'ordinary life.'

Turner-Crowson (1993) puts the issue this way:

> *Evidence . . . shows that the DGH model tends to undermine effective integration between psychiatric in-patient and community services, whilst enhancing the less important integration of in-patient psychiatry with other DGH surgical and medical specialties. (p 9)*

Thus the argument for separating mental health services from the acute hospital and linking them as well as care for dementia patients along with other services for the elderly, in separate community trusts, as many now are, turns not so much on their clinical similarities or the advantages in terms of shared facilities, but rather the management advantages of having one organisation or team serving that client group.

On this analysis, the key factors determining clusters of activity are not clinical links of the kind defined in the previous chapter but rather a much wider range of connections between services distributed over a wide area which are important for a particular group of users. In other words, in contrast to the emphasis on links between hospital specialists, the emphasis is on links between specialists outside the hospital including professionals who are not clinicians, such as social service or voluntary organisation staff specialising in the care of particular groups of patients.

Within the framework set out in Chapter 2, the argument rests on different views of where economies of scope lie, within the hospital or elsewhere, and over which groups of activities. In the case of children, for example, the argument for offering psychiatric services to children along with other paediatric services within acute general hospitals is primarily based on the desirability of children's services themselves being integrated. This in turn stems from the fact that many diseases are specific to the younger age groups and that children have distinct physiological characteristics; hence it is beneficial, in terms of quality of care, to specialise across the age group rather than type of disease or part of the body as with most specialties.

To conclude: the potential for separating out certain of the existing functions of the acute general hospital is clear. However, a simple listing of functions does not assist with the next stage of determining whether they should all be carried out within alternative clusters, also called hospitals, or whether they have so little in common that they can be dispersed to all manner of locations. Looking at the list set out in Table 3.1, it would appear that the interactions between most separable functions is likely to be minimal, both in terms of personnel and equipment, and many can be carried out in a range of settings, intermediate institution, GP surgery or even the home.

Whether the potential for separation should be realised is another matter. In particular, the cost implications of separation have yet to be taken into account. In some countries, the free-standing surgical centre is common. In others, free-standing diagnostic facilities are found. It may be inferred, from their financial viability, that such facilities can provide services at competitive cost. But within the UK context, no evidence for that is available. Thus it is easier to demonstrate the potential for some functions now carried out in district general hospitals to be dispersed to other settings than to show what benefits arise from doing so.

Specialist Functions

Broadly, these are of two types. Specialties such as neurosciences, in which there are only a small number of consultant posts in the country as a whole, and specialised units within larger specialties such as cancer which deal with the relatively uncommon types of the disease. While the scale of such activities dictates that they cannot be found on all the sites where the bulk of acute hospital activities takes place, do they need to be located at some of these sites or can they be free-standing? In other words, do they also enjoy economies of scope?

Most recent reviews of specialised services endorse the advantages of being located near to other specialties, reflecting the arguments for clustering set out in the previous chapter. Thus the London Burns and Plastic Service Review suggests that the treatment of patients with major burns is best provided:

- *on an acute hospital site with other surgical specialties with which plastic surgeons work as some patients with major burns are suffering from major trauma or other serious injuries*
- *where there is ready access to paediatricians (as burns and scalds often occur in childhood) and renal physicians (as burns hypovolaemic shock can occasionally result in renal failure)*
- *where patients are cared for by specialist teams led by plastic surgeons and anaesthetists*
- *by nursing staff with a wide range of skills – e.g. ENB 264, ITU, RSCN, as appropriate – and a full spectrum of health and social care professionals – e.g. physiotherapists, occupational therapists, dieticians and social workers*
- *where there is a separate burns theatre*
- *where there is a combined intensive care/high dependency area with access to low dependency beds where patients with major burns recovering after skin grafting and patients with minor burns can be nursed. (Rehabilitation after wound healing is a prolonged process and some of these patients may require a degree of support from many disciplines at an early stage that can only be reasonably provided in hospital)*
- *where there is a full range of pathology services – particularly bacteriology, biochemistry and blood transfusion – readily available for acute, complex multi-system disorders*
- *from sites which maximise access for patients, their relatives and others because of the lengthy time many patients spend in burn units. (para 87)*

If these arguments are accepted, but if access considerations rule out the 'maximum scope' hospital, then differences in roles between general hospitals must emerge. But exactly what those differences should be still remains to be determined.

In the case of services such as cancer or cardiology, such differences are usually expressed in terms of a hierarchy. Thus, the Expert Review of Cancer Services (Department of Health, 1994) describes a system of cancer care based on Cancer Centres and Cancer Units, as follows:

Designated Cancer Units should be created in many district general hospitals. These should be of a size to support clinical teams with sufficient expertise and facilities to manage the commoner cancers.

Designated Cancer Centres should provide expertise in the management of all cancers, including common cancers within their immediate geographical locality and less common cancers by referral from Cancer Units. They will provide specialist diagnostic and therapeutic techniques including radiotherapy. (p 7)

Other service reviews have produced similar structures. But while the notion of a hierarchy can be seen as the obvious response to the need to balance considerations of access against the benefits of specialisation, it is by no means a precise notion. In the case of cardiac services, for example, the British Cardiac Society (1993) sets out four options, representing different ways of determining the role of specialist centres:

- *That district hospital cardiologists should undertake no invasive work and refer all cases to specialist centres for investigation.*
- *That district hospital cardiologists with appropriate training be offered specified sessions at the specialist centre for invasive investigation mainly of an elective nature.*
- *That some district hospitals, particularly those that are geographically disadvantaged, develop facilities for invasive investigation. This may be in conjunction with neighbouring districts to ensure that expensive facilities are used with utmost efficiency and will require that appropriate skills are developed and maintained in all members of the team.*
- *That elective invasive investigation in district hospitals should become the norm and that specialist centres concentrate their resources in the development of interventional techniques, provision of emergency treatments, and provision of diagnostic services for their own catchment population only. (p 4)*

Thus in this particular area of work, there are several ways in which advantages of scale can be realised. Furthermore, the nature of those advantages may change. As the British Cardiac Society puts it:

The dividing line between the services that should be provided in every district hospital and those that should be provided in specialised, so-called tertiary centres, is always likely to vary and will depend on local facilities and local skills. (p 3)

Similarly, the case of cancer care – see Table 3.2 – the role of the various tiers are far from distinct. Only three – radiotherapy, second opinions, joint tumours etc. – are reserved for the 'highest' or most specialised tiers. Others may be provided outside the hospital itself.

The extent of local provision for any one service itself turns on how the balance between access and clinical quality is determined for other services. Thus, if the arguments for concentration and clustering those specialties of central importance for emergency care are given greater weight, that would reduce the case for other services to be supplied in other

Table 3.2 Cancer services: division of function between hospitals and other providers

Service	Community	GP	Local DGH	Larger DGH	Cancer Centre
Diagnostic	−	+	+	+	+
Surgery					
Diagnostic	−	−	+	+	+
Therapy	−	−	−	+	+
Radiotherapy	−	−	−	−	+
Chemotherapy	−	−	−	+	+
Supportive care	+	+	+	+	+
Palliative care	+	+	+	+	+
Second opinion	−	−	−	−	+
Joint tumour management, ENT, gynae, ortho, paediatric etc	−	−	−	−	+
Screening	+	+	+	+	+
Prevention	+	+	+	+	+

Source: Sikora and Waxman (1993)

hospitals. In other words, the greater the scale of the hospital, the more it can provide some specialised services in-house. But, at the same time, it would increase the case for separating out functions not vital to emergency care into intermediate institutions.

Thus the hospital serving some 0.5 to 0.7 million people – a proposal in the Oxford Strategy – would be large enough to allow specialisation in services such as ophthalmology which could only be achieved within a network of smaller DGHs, by some form of specialisation between them. But a hospital of this size would, outside the conurbations, be inaccessible for many, so the case for local hospitals or intermediate institutions providing a restricted range of services would increase.

As far as the highly specialised services are concerned, ie those serving national or regional catchment populations, most clinical reviews support their location in a general hospital. In the case of cancer services, the London Review explicitly considered the case for a free-standing centre and rejected it, in these terms, while noting that the largest treatment centre for cancer in the country, the Christie in Manchester, is a single specialty site:

Our conclusion is that this is not the pattern of care that should be the preferred model for the future, for the following reasons:

Cancer services are concerned with the care of acutely ill patients, for whom direct access, on site, to general and specialist physicians and surgeons is very desirable. Most cancer patients are older people needing a wide range of other expertise from medical and paramedical staff, as do other elderly patients.

The general diagnostic and support services for cancer, such as pathology and imaging, are required just as much for patients who do not have cancer, as for those who do. Duplication of such expensive services is quite wrong in both equipment and manpower terms. Equally, it is desirable that the specialists who work in this field should maintain a breadth of diagnostic expertise from a mix of medical cases, which should not and does not prevent their own development of special interests in cancers or in other fields.

New developments in radiotherapy equipment, for instance, multi-lead collimators are now already being tested in several Centres in the UK. This dispersed pattern of innovation has we believe been a strength of the NHS. There seems no special reason why such testing should in future be restricted to any one Centre, which would not necessarily have the expertise in its staff for any particular specialised development. This would in any case be against a 'market philosophy', as exemplified by the links which some departments already have which assist manufacturers to the NHS.

New developments in molecular medicine and genetics, whilst they strike at the very causes of cancer, and hence hold real hope of advances in prevention and treatment, are also of great significance for many other medical and surgical conditions; inflammatory bowel disease, asthma and diabetes for example. It is, we are advised, essential that these research developments are exploited in association with the research environment of general medical services, not cancer alone.

Staff in training, whether in medical, paramedical or supporting services do we believe learn best within the broad environment of general acute services, rather than by working wholly in a specialist hospital. (pp 51-52)

Most reviews come to similar conclusions, but in doing so they take only one specialty at a time. That leads to the question of whether all specialised functions should themselves be clustered together. The case for doing so has been put forward in relation to trauma (Templeton 1994). This case is based on the presumed advantage of 'comprehensive back-up in all specialities' in the treatment of very severely injured patients. The idea of a trauma centre is currently being evaluated so the advantages of this degree of clustering remain to be demonstrated. If it proved to be worthwhile and changes in hospital structures made accordingly, that would lead to a two-tier hierarchy for emergency care with the upper tier consisting of some 20 or so hospitals in the whole of England. But that would still leave open the division of roles based on specialisation in other areas within the second tier, for which the same degree of clustering is not required as may be justified for severely injured patients. Is it important or immaterial, for example, for cancer centres to be located in the same hospital as other specialised facilities, such as cardiac, or any other specialty within which different degrees of specialisation are required?

No agreed way of defining the importance of different clusters exists. The York Health Economics Consortium (Ryder *et al*, undated) has devised a system of weighting the connections between specialties on a simple scale, a small extract from which is shown in Table 3.3. The weights assist in distinguishing *prima facie* which options are likely to make sense, but they are not refined enough to identify which groups of patients would do better or worse in different clusters. Neither do the 'desired' lists of specialties typically cited in professional reviews, some of which are cited in the notes to this chapter.

Table 3.3 Clinical priorities – 'combined' inter-specialty links matrix

		1	2	3	4	5	6
1	Accident & Emergency		0	3	3	3	1
2	Accident & Emergency Child	0		3	0	0	1
3	Intensive Therapy Unit	0	0		1	2	1
4	Cancer Care Unit	0	0	2		3	3
5	General Medicine	0	0	3	3		2
6	Cardiology	0	0	3	3	1	

Source: Ryder *et al.* (undated)

As a result, there is no clear way of determining how important the co-existence of particular groups of specialties is. It would be reasonable to assume, as for trauma care, that certain groups may be important for some patients, but not necessarily for others. If those who do not benefit incur access costs or other penalties, then here too trade-offs between different groups of patients will exist.

3.2 Routes to Hospital

Once hospitals specialise, then how patients are allocated to, or choose between, hospitals has to be considered. In some cases, this is straightforward enough: the general practitioner chooses the consultant most appropriate to the needs of the patient. But in others, it may not be correct, as a recent report from the Royal Colleges of General Practice and of Psychiatry (1995) has shown for those patients with medical symptoms not explained by any disease. This concluded that a significant proportion of patients being referred to district general hospitals had psychological rather than physiological conditions, which were not being detected.

Routing within the hospital system may also be inappropriate. The Audit Commission (1994b) refers, in respect of hospital services for children, to:

> largely historical referral patterns which can result in routine conditions being treated at expensive regional centres, while more complex surgery is attempted at district level. (p 45)

Similarly, the London Neurosciences Review notes that:

> one of the past failings of the tertiary centre has been 'failure' to ensure that the patient returns as infrequently as possible to the centre. (para 61)

As the inverted commas indicate, failure may be deliberate. But in other cases, incorrect allocation may arise from poor information. GPs may not know who among a team of orthopaedic surgeons is best suited to carry out a particular procedure. That difficulty might be met by making referrals to departments rather than individuals. Alternatively, ways must be found of making the requisite information available, whether that be through private initiative, as with the *Directory of Breast Cancer Services* (King's Fund, 1995). The need for the *Directory* arose from the perception that women were not receiving appropriate care precisely because the 'routing' system was poor.

In respect of elective surgery, the South East Thames Region report assumes that the division of roles between main and local facility would be based on agreed protocols. The Oxford Strategy assumes that individual surgeons will decide whether or not they can operate in local hospitals without immediate access to intensive care facilities. Both may work, but the former are far from straightforward in practice (McKee and Clarke, 1995), and the merits of the latter currently have to be taken on trust since no evidence is routinely available on the clinical outcomes of operating in different settings.

As far as emergency care is concerned, the general hospital can be seen as a device for simplifying routing decisions outside the hospital itself by presenting a single option for patients and health care workers outside it. As a consequence of that simplification, however, it may receive work that is not appropriate to it, ie conditions which are not serious even though they appear to be.

The task of distinguishing the two could be seen as a key function of the human and physical resources available in the hospital. That implicitly assumes that such distinctions cannot be made outside the hospital itself, but that assumption may be wrong. At one end of the scale, the argument is sometimes put against developing local minor injuries units that people would not recognise the limits of what it could be and would waste time going to it when they should be seeking treatment elsewhere. Experience suggests (personal communication) that in general practice people can make the appropriate distinctions, but they may not always do so. At the other end of the scale, where serious injuries occur, ambulance crews may be faced with the choice of taking casualties to the nearest hospital, or deciding to go elsewhere. Though their experience is greater than the average patient, they can nevertheless be faced with dilemmas which they are not equipped to resolve themselves. If they take seriously ill patients to the 'wrong' hospital, then on-referral must be arranged, possibly causing delay. If they take everyone to the best equipped, then they incur unnecessary journey costs. The former error creates risks to patients, the latter is inefficient.

Routing decisions for emergency care still largely follow established patterns ie to the nearest hospital. But, as noted below, developments in information technology are beginning to create new options which draw on the knowledge-base which the general hospital commands, while not physically involving the hospital at all. As these examples indicate, once hospitals carry out different roles, the single district general hospital represents only part of a larger system within which signposts may be required to ensure that patients end up in the right place. However, more may be at stake than information. Within the hierarchical model, the cancer patient is served not so much by a hospital as by a service running across several. The next question we consider is how, in such a system, services and hospitals should relate to each other.

3.3 Relations between hospitals

Within the 'old' NHS all the hospitals in a district were managed by the health authority. The creation of trusts has not essentially changed that. There are no hospital chains in the UK and the question of whether a trust can establish a hospital outside its old district boundary is moot. Within the old system and to a large extent the existing one, relationships between hospitals, where these are not managed as part of a single group, are based on the professional one of referral: patients are 'passed on,' usually with a transfer of clinical responsibility but sometimes with shared responsibility, to another hospital more appropriate to their needs. The transfer may be done in haste, in the case of an emergency, or at a more leisurely pace when a further opinion is sought.

However, a number of proposals have emerged from the London specialty reviews which imply close links between hospitals – in different trusts – within the hub and spoke model. It is already established practice for 'large' hospitals to provide services to smaller ones. Surgical teams used to take it in turn to visit a smaller unit, within the same district. Now, that unit may be part of a separate organisation. If the arrangement continues, then in effect the receiving unit is the provider of a basic infrastructure into which other services can plug. What this means within the terms of our analysis is that the service is a more important unit of analysis than the hospital. The hub and spoke model suggests the same. If the links between specialties in different institutions are more important than those between specialties of different types within the same institution, how should the inter-institutional links be made?

In the case of the Neurosciences Review, (London Implementation Group, 1993g) the nature of the link is put in professional terms:

> *Medical, nursing and therapy staff appointed to district general hospital departments will have professional links with the clinical neuroscience centre in order to ensure that their expertise is maintained and developed over time and in the case of senior medical staff that link must be contractual. (p 64)*

As for linkages between hubs and spokes:

> *A seamless service can be achieved by establishing formal linkages between the (tertiary/referral) centre, the district general hospital and the wider primary, community and social care services. (para 52)*

As far as the hospital end of this spectrum is concerned, the Review suggests that:

> *An important element of the service is that the tertiary centre should become an accredited or preferred supplier within the internal market ... This model can only be successful if the contractual relationship between purchaser, secondary provider and tertiary provider is linked. That linkage should preferably be through a long term contractual relationship to ensure the best use of capital investment. (para 54)*

Similarly, the Cardiac Review (London Implementation Group, 1993c) affirmed the establishment of close links between tertiary and secondary centres as an important professional priority and that that should consist of joint appointments, rotation of staff, collaboration in research and joint clinical audit.

How far should this contractual relationship be taken? Already in some areas, some services are provided within a number of hospitals by a single group of clinicians and support staff some of whom are rotated between sites. But there are other possibilities. The London Review of Renal Services (London Implementation Group, 1993f) suggested three:

1. *Minimal care facilities managed by the 'base' renal unit both medically and administratively. In many instances these have been 'free-standing' and have had no links with local hospitals.*
2. *Satellite renal units set up within district general hospitals and managed administratively as a part of that district general hospital.*
3. *Satellite renal units contracted out to the private sector.*

The implication of this approach is that the specialty or client group is the critical unit of organisation, and the general hospital becomes a basic infrastructure into which the full range of specialties can fit. The specialty might be focused on a single specialty hospital, or be part of a larger establishment. Either way, the model of the hospital as an integrated single site management structure is undermined. When relations with providers outside the hospital system are taken into account, the subversion may be taken further, as the next chapter makes clear.

3.4 Conclusion

Many functions currently carried out within acute general hospitals do not need to be done in one and the same institution. At the simpler end of the scale, a wide range of activities may be dispersed at no clinical risk, but whether that would be beneficial on cost and access grounds and how they should be clustered in intermediate institutions can only be judged in the light of local geography, the availability of buildings and so on. Separation of other activities such as elective surgery or maternity care may impose risks, so whether this is desirable depends in part on how well any risks can be anticipated and in part on the preferences of patients.

At the other end of the scale, the need for hospitals to take on different roles follows from differences between specialties, particularly the different catchment areas which they require. However, there is no established way of determining groupings of specialised services. The specialty reviews cited in this chapter and other similar reviews identify the significant linkages for their service. But the advantages these links offer vary from ease of communications to the long term advantages that may result from links between clinical activity and research. Their relative importance is, therefore, not easy to assess: the reviews themselves do not attempt to do so.

The task of evaluating this wide range of effects is complicated enough; the task becomes yet more difficult when the role of the hospital is considered in the context of the health care system as a whole. This is the subject of the next chapter.

CHAPTER 4

Hospitals and other providers

Underlying the argument so far is the assumption that hospitals and other care providers have distinct roles. In the UK, that is generally true. To oversimplify, the general practitioner, usually the patient's first point of contact with the health service, deals with the majority of cases, perhaps drawing on the analytic resources of the hospital for advice, and gate-keeps access to specialist services within the hospital. Community services provide support after, or in the case of maternity services before and after, hospital care.

Oversimplification though this may be, there has been since the foundation of the NHS a sharp separation of roles between hospitals and other providers. The reasons for this lie largely in the organisation of care within the NHS, rather than its content: in other countries, patients have direct access to specialists based in hospitals or with access to hospital facilities. In the UK, they do not.

Even within this framework, however, in some areas roles can and do overlap. Hospital accident and emergency departments carry out a large amount of work which could easily be carried out by a GP or a practice nurse: estimates vary as to its extent, but figures of 30–40 per cent are often quoted (Dale, 1992).

The response to emergency is only one area, however, where the role of the hospital may actually or potentially overlap with that of other providers and hence substitution between them may be feasible. In many areas, however, hospitals and other providers work collaboratively rather than competitively; consultation with a GP may lead to a consultation with a hospital specialist and a hospital stay. As a consequence, improvement in the quality of service offered by general practitioners and others working outside the hospital may lead to the identification of demands of the sort that, as things now stand, only hospitals can provide. In these circumstances, their roles are complementary rather than competitive.

We then consider a third form of relationship, diversion. Within the UK health care system the hospital depends for the vast majority of its work on other care providers. The gate-keeping role of general practice is a system of demand management for the hospital over which it has no control within the current structure of health services. In principle, general practice deals with cases that do not need the specialist services of the hospital and hence avoids, or at least reduces, their inappropriate use. But its role might go further. The scope for health promotion and preventive care is increasingly being emphasised. If successful, this role can lead to a reduction in the volume of work with which hospitals, as well as other providers, have to deal.

The first part of this chapter considers these different forms of relationship between hospitals and other providers; the second looks briefly at the implications for hospital organisation.

4.1 Types of relationship

Where overlaps occur, there is clearly scope for substitution. In some cases the overlap and hence area of substitution are because roles are ill-defined and hence inappropriate use occurs. For example, there is evidence that once patients are referred to hospital outpatient clinics, they attend more often subsequently than there is need for them to do. Hospital use in these cases is inappropriate either because there is no clinical benefit to such patients or because what is required can be done by a GP. A study of rheumatology clinics (Sullivan and Hoare, 1990) found that a high proportion of patients made four or more visits but this could not be accounted for by the severity of their disease or diagnoses. It appeared that junior doctors did not have the experience or confidence to refer patients back to their GPs.

Similarly, there is evidence that hospital inpatient facilities are sometimes not used appropriately even where the reason for admission is valid: a number of surveys have found that people were being kept in unnecessarily, sometimes because of failure to implement proper discharge procedures, in others because of lack of suitable facilities to discharge patients to. Such inappropriate use can be large. A study in Oxford (Anderson *et al*, 1989) suggested that only 38 per cent of the bed days of the patients studied did have medical, nursing or life support reasons for being in a provincial teaching hospital bed. Other studies (Pearson, 1994), however, have produced smaller figures and of course there is every reason to expect variation from hospital to hospital and from one year to another.

In these cases, it may be said that hospital facilities are misused, and hence that some of the existing workload should be transferred to other settings such as intermediate institutions or the patient's own home and in the extreme case not done at all.

If inappropriate use of these kinds were eliminated, the result might be a small reduction in the level of hospital provision, but no more than that. More important is the question of whether work now deemed to be appropriate to the hospital can be handled better or at least as well in other settings, which may or may not be called hospitals, but which would be different to the present structure of provision.

In thinking about the scope and nature of substitution, it helps to make a number of distinctions. In some cases, the essential shift is one of location: the same activity may take place in other settings, eg pre-testing and prior consultation may be carried out by the same consultant but in a different location such as a health centre or GP surgery. Similarly, accelerated discharge and rehabilitation may be provided by hospital nursing staff working in the community through hospital outreach. The locus of care changes but the managerial and professional responsibility may not. We term this *spatial substitution*.

In other cases, however, the whole episode of care may be handled without recourse to specialised hospital facilities at all, either at home, in the GP surgery, or in inter-mediate facilities under the control of the GP. We term this *mode substitution*, ie the same need is served in a different way just as a transport need may be served by road, rail or air.

To define the scope for substitution, the components of a hospital stay need to be distinguished. A stay in hospital, even a short one, consists of a large number of elements, involving contributions from a large number of professionals. Studies of the interactions of patients with hospital staff show that they may involve some 30 to 40 different people, most of whom are offering a distinct contribution to the overall care episode. Some of these may have to occur within the confines of the hospital but not all.

Perhaps the most straightforward example is the period immediately after an operation. In the vast majority of cases, after a short period immediately following the operation, patients may only require nursing care. Hospital-at-home schemes focusing on early discharge in effect relocate that element of the stay to another place – the patient's home – and replace the hospital nurse with one working in the community. In this instance, substitution of part of a care episode has occurred.

Once the possibility of substitution is acknowledged, it is helpful to talk in terms of modes of care. A mode will have some 'markets' in which it is dominant – in the case of hospitals, intensive care facilities and expensive diagnostic equipment and some characteristics peculiar to it, which distinguish it from others. Some characteristics, however, will be contingent, not inherent: they can be altered through appropriate management action. Thus, as a matter of fact, only hospitals may have access to certain diagnostic equipment, but that could be changed through appropriate investment in mobile facilities.

With the exception of some accident and emergency care, hospitals in the UK system form part of a 'mixed mode' since most hospital care episodes begin with the GP surgery and many end with it or with a community nursing service. In terms of logic it would be correct, if linguistically cumbersome, to infer that any difference in the way that care is provided could be said to create a different mode. Cumbersome though it may be to think in terms of multiple modes of care, careful examination of any particular service or care group will reveal different ways of combining human and physical resources to do more or less the same job. It is a matter of convenience what they are called.

The possibility of mode or spatial substitution does not, however, eliminate the basic trade-offs between cost, quality and access. In terms of the framework for analysis set out in Chapter 2, providers outside hospital in areas where substitution is feasible may offer better access – in the extreme case no access costs because services are provided at home. The issue then is whether this advantage has to be paid for in terms of higher cost or reduced quality. If access were given an infinite weight then it would be feasible to spatially substitute most hospital services, eg through mobile operating theatres, and in this way revert, if in slightly more hygienic form, to the 19th century version of acute care on the kitchen table. For the individual – unless of course that individual is a head of state – that would appear profligate of resources but whether it would be profligate for otherwise isolated populations is another matter.

However, once different modes of treatment enter the picture, the trade-offs become more complicated than has been implied so far. For simplicity it has been assumed that in thinking about choices between different kinds of hospital, user views, access apart, could be ignored since the 'care experience' would be the same for each variant. But people may prefer different styles of treatment which are peculiar to each mode. They may prefer, for example, to be treated in an intermediate institution, not simply because of the access advantage but also because they prefer the physical environment it offers or the continuity of personnel which a smaller institution can offer. As a result, quality becomes a much more complicated notion than has been recognised so far, since it may embody any facet of the patient's experience of care which they like or dislike.

It follows that the concept of substitution is neither purely a clinical nor a financial one: it is also a matter of choice or preference on the part of the service user. It follows also that the boundary between hospital and services elsewhere should be blurred: it is not all or nothing. The principle of hospital use minimisation set out in the 1962 Plan and other official documents is therefore too strong, assuming as it does a clear cut division of function. Equally, so is the counter principle that care must be provided as close to home as possible, which begs the question of the weight to be given to cost – if that is higher – and quality – if that is lower – in the home or near home environment. Instead the principle should be rephrased in terms of 'optimal balance' (Hughes and Gordon, 1992). That balance may depend on patient choice as much as on technical considerations for even within a given service such as maternity, different users, in objectively the same circumstances, may make different choices if they are given the opportunity. Furthermore, it does not imply a once and for all solution. On the contrary, relative costs and preferences may vary over time: any balance is temporary and prone to change.

If areas of potential substitution are seen, as they would be for other goods and services, as areas of competition, then there is no reason why the shift should be all in one direction. At present, the emphasis in government policy statements is on shifts away from hospitals, primarily because the scope for delivering what was traditionally hospital care by other modes is becoming apparent. But changes in medical technology and changes in the way that hospital-based services are provided may offer opportunities for moves in the other direction.

The distinction between primary and secondary services tends to blur when different modes are taken into account. It still makes sense to talk about points of first contact – usually primary care but also, in the case of emergency facilities, hospitals – and to distinguish between acute conditions needing immediate response and others which can be deferred without serious risk. But these distinctions need not be mirrored in sharp divisions in the organisation and management of services as they are now. It becomes feasible, for example, to think in terms of an emergency response which is based in an intermediate facility, provided by district nurses and managed by a hospital-based consultant. This may serve part of the market which is typically served by the emergency facilities of the hospital or that normally covered by general practice or both. Similarly, a general practitioner may, as some hospitals have found, usefully be located within the hospital emergency facility.

In most spheres of economic life, the mix of resources actually chosen would be influenced by, on the provider side, changes in costs of the relevant resources and changes in the available technology, and, on the user side, the preferences of users for different forms of service or, in our terminology, modes of delivery. Within most health care systems, particularly that obtaining in the UK, the scope for substitution has not been actively pursued because the roles of different organisations and professions have been defined by historical circumstance and relative professional power. As a result, the process of defining different modes of care delivery across the whole spectrum has not been systematically addressed and hence its potential not been fully identified. How great that might be is discussed in Chapter 8.

While total substitution is feasible for some care, most care involving hospitals is part of a longer episode involving other providers of care: the various providers complement each other. In the case of some patients such as those with diabetes, those links between hospitals and other care providers may be open-ended, extending in time to the end of the patient's life. In other circumstances, such as patients needing home-based care after an inpatient stay, they need to be in place for only a short period. In both cases, an increase in work within primary care – in these cases the initial identification of the need for treatment, be it on an episodic or continuing basis – leads to an increase in the work of the hospital.

Nevertheless the Government appears to assume, in promoting a switch to primary care, that improvements to primary and community health service will reduce the use of hospitals. In some cases this may be so: Farmer and Coulter (1990) found that use of hospital facilities by diabetic patients was lower in well-organised general practices. Similarly, the more patients understand their own conditions, the greater the chances of reducing emergency admission. Osman *et al* (1994) found that patients with severe asthmatic conditions had fewer admissions after an enhanced education programme than a control group.

But the reverse may also be true. A general practitioner may fail in whole or part to identify the appropriate response either through incomplete or inaccurate diagnosis or lack of familiarity with what hospitals can offer. The need for surgery or inpatient treatment may not be recognised. A better-trained and informed practitioner may therefore pass on more cases than one who is less well informed. In this case, the relationship continues to be one of complementarity: better primary or preventive care leads to greater hospital use by identifying more cases for treatment than would otherwise have been identified. This effect has emerged from studies of the care of children: one study (Durojaiye *et al*, 1989) in the Nottingham Health District tracing the growth in the numbers of children admitted to hospital found that improvements in primary care over the period of the study, 1975 to 1985, had not resulted in fewer admissions.

Similarly, complementarity and substitution, while opposite effects, in practice lie closely together. In some cases, protocols define the role of all the professionals involved. Using these, shifts between different modes of care may take place, not through a rejection of one mode for another, but through a redefinition of the work of the hospital-based doctor in relation to the general practitioner or community nurse, or vice versa. Thus substitution may take place within what is essentially a complementary relationship.

In some cases, action may be taken in the community which will prevent or reduce the load on the hospital by eliminating the need for care entirely. Preventive and health promotion measures fall into this category; if they are effective they eliminate or reduce the need for hospital as well as other forms of care.

However, the impact of preventive measures is more complicated than that way of putting it implies. In the short run, measures such as screening for cancer or other diseases can increase the workload on the hospital by identifying cases for urgent and expensive intervention. Subsequently, the workload may reduce but after that a further, third round effect, may occur: diseases are themselves substitutes for each other. A different type of demand may emerge at a later date. The same is true of measures designed to promote health by reducing the risks of particular diseases developing. Elimination, in other words, is rarely total. Usually, it combines elements both of substitution and complementarity, once its effects over time are taken into account.

To conclude: identification of the different general relationship between hospitals and other providers helps to define the various ways in which they may interact. But it does nothing to establish their relative importance; how that may be done is considered in Chapter 8.

4.2 Implications for hospital structures

At the heart of the analysis set out in Chapters 2 and 3 was an emphasis on linkages between the human and physical resources which a hospital commands; it was these which justified the concept of the general hospital. But there are important links too between services within and services outside hospital. In some instances, these may be very straightforward and short-lived: a patient may have a given procedure carried out in a day case unit and subsequently a visual check may be desirable on the healing process. Once that is done and the check finds nothing untoward, the care episode is complete.

But other care episodes are much more drawn out and indeed, in the case of chronic conditions, may be indefinite. In these cases patients may pass from one responsible professional to another, and in some cases, back and forth between them. The aim of policy in these circumstances is often put in terms of seamlessness, which means that the patient should not be aware of the fact that different providers are involved. The appropriate unit of analysis is the care process as a whole. The logic may be taken further: in the case of care for particular groups of patients, it may be the programme or client group.

As already noted in the case of mental health, this has already been widely accepted. Whereas, in the 1960s, the critical connections appeared to be between different hospital specialists within the general hospital, now they appear to be between specialists of various kinds, some within NHS provider units, some in other settings, be these local authority run, privately managed or by a voluntary organisation.

A similar case can be made for services to children. Children, particularly younger ones, are in continuous contact with the health services, not only for acute care, and the wide range of childhood diseases and illnesses, but also for screening and surveillance, for which a structured programme is provided. Twenty years ago, the Court Report (1976) suggested that services to children should be provided on an integrated basis across all providers, including general practitioners specialising in paediatric care. As the Audit Commission report *Seen but not Heard* (1994) indicated, such integration remains a long way off and the obstacles are severe, in large part because different providers are involved.

If a case can be made in terms of the needs of the client group for unifying responsibility across all providers, the question is whether the organisation of the hospital should reflect this and whether the kind of relationship suggested in the hub and spoke model be extended to include services outside the hospital itself. As Robinson (1994) has put it:

> *Shall the coordination of care be performed by the hospital staff, through diversification into related services, or by some other organizational entity, which relates to the hospital through contracts rather than unified ownership? (p 273)*

If the service – be it paediatrics, renal care or any other where close links between hospitals and other providers are required – were managed from outside the hospital itself, then the hospital would cease to be an integrated management structure. Rather it would be a common user facility, analogous to an electricity grid or a transport interchange.

Such a structure is easiest to grasp for the intermediate facility, be it community or local hospital. The clinical links between the various activities appropriate to such settings may be weak, but there may be other advantages in grouping them together, in terms of sharing support facilities and other common services, and enabling professionals from different organisations to form more effective working relationships. In this sense, the building, its management and support structure can readily be seen as a general health facility into which a range of functions may be packed which may be provided by a number of different providers.

This way of looking at the large acute hospital is less familiar and indeed it runs against the current trend towards integrating management structures. But division of acute general hospitals in this way is not unknown: in some cases, it has developed as a result of the divisions created between acute and community units when trusts were established by dividing up organisations using the same facilities. In these circumstances, normal clinical relations within the hospital, eg when patients need to be transferred to intensive care from long-stay facilities, still operate but across a contractual and organisational divide.

But even if the service or care group might be a better unit of organisation and analysis than the hospital, that does not have any necessary bearing on the central issues considered in Chapter 2. Suppose that recognition of the need for integration across providers led to the creation of a paediatric service organised from outside the hospital but employing hospital-based personnel. Even if that form of service organisation had merit, it would still leave the basic argument for clustering the work of hospital paediatricians alongside other hospital-based clinicians.

In practice, however, as Malcolm (1990) has argued in relation to New Zealand, a change of organisational structure may be important. A service structure, by transcending the physical boundaries of the hospital as it now stands, may facilitate locational and mode substitution by removing boundaries implicit in organisational structures.

4.3 Conclusion

This and the previous two chapters have set out a wide range of arguments bearing on the central questions posed in Chapter 1:

- how many hospitals should there be?
- what should each be doing?

Taking hospitals by themselves, the key planning issue is to find the right balance between the benefits of access as against the benefits of clustering and concentration – scope and scale – and the costs of achieving different configurations.

If the possibility of substitution by other providers is introduced, then the prior issue is: what are the services which hospitals are best qualified to supply? It follows that the questions of what is the best pattern of hospital provision and what is the right balance between hospital and other forms of provision are inextricably linked. Although the framework based on quality, cost and access remains central to thinking about alternative dispositions of resources, instead of one set of trade-offs, there are many such sets.

In order to get the best pattern of service delivery requires, therefore, estimates of the costs and benefits of a vast number of alternative dispositions of resources in the health care system as a whole and, within those dispositions, alternative ways of organising them. That task is too large to attempt here. Instead, the following three chapters focus on the central themes of quality, cost and access for the hospital itself.

CHAPTER 5

Scale, scope and clinical quality

Although the district general hospital was intended to raise the quality of care, the link between staffing and facilities on the one hand and quality of care on the other was assumed rather than demonstrated. No system of monitoring or audit was established to test whether that assumption was justified, so as a result, there is no routine data to call on which would in retrospect show whether the district general hospital performed better than the single specialty hospital, whether the quality of care it provided met with some externally agreed standards, or whether large units perform better than small, even in those areas such as maternity care or minor surgery where there are different modes of provision in different parts of the country. Essentially that remains true now: although following the NHS and Community Care Act 1990, systems of medical audit are in place throughout the NHS, they do not provide indicators of performance for hospitals doing the same things but with different clinical configurations. Published or readily available evidence on different patterns of provision in different parts of the country do not shed light on the merits of different forms of hospital organisation.

The evidence presented in this chapter comes, therefore, from *ad hoc* studies of two main kinds: first, statistical studies of the relationship between hospital characteristics and clinical quality, and second, reviews, typically by a group of clinicians working in one specialty, either of the quality of care achieved in particular instances or of the human and physical resources required to achieve a 'high' level of clinical quality. Their findings are considered in the first two parts of this chapter. In the final part, some data are presented on the current pattern of clinical activity.

5.1 Research studies

A number of studies have been carried out which attempt to relate the actual quality or outcome of treatment to the volume of activity either within the hospital as a whole or in the execution of a particular procedure. The definition of quality is usually a narrow one – typically it is based purely on mortality rates during hospital stays or within 30 days of discharge. According to a survey by Black and Johnston (1990):

It appears that hospital volume is associated with the effectiveness of some health services (most surgery, cardiac catheterisation, trauma care) and may be of importance in other areas (neonatal care, coronary care, burn care). (p 111)

The cautious wording reflects the imperfect data which the various studies reviewed relied on and the methodological difficulties involved in analysing them. The authors go on to point out that the observed relationship could rest on a number of different factors:

Some of the limitations of the literature on volume:outcome will be all too apparent. Firstly, it ignores some areas of hospital care because of difficulties in measuring case-mix and outcome. Secondly [their] review has deliberately been made to assess the impact of volume on the effectiveness of care. No attempt has been made to assess the impact of volume on the humanity, equity or efficiency of service . . . thirdly, most studies restrict their measurement of effectiveness to case-fatality. This latter point is particularly important where studies use, as most do, mortality within the hospital, rather than within 30 days of discharge. A hospital might for instance score well by discharging people who die soon afterwards. (p 111)

Another and more detailed survey (Luft *et al*, 1990) also found that while a majority of studies confirmed the existence of a volume:outcome relationship, some studies had not found one. Their own work, taking 12 procedure groups and data from 150 hospitals, did find such a relationship for all except one procedure group. In some cases the relationship appeared to continue indefinitely as volume rose, in others it tailed off above a threshold. The results are shown in Table 5.1.

The Table shows the excess deaths in small hospitals, ie the difference between the actual number and the number which would have occurred had the outcomes been the same as large hospitals – after allowing in principle for patient characteristics. In some cases such as open heart surgery, this difference is large in relation to the total death rate; in others such as biliary tract surgery, quite small.

Another survey (Office of Technology Assessment, 1988), concluded as follows:

In summary, the available studies reviewed by OTA provide rather substantial evidence that worse outcomes occur at lower volumes for most of the procedures and diagnoses that has-been studied. However, the volume-outcome relationship is not universal. For stomach operations and fractures of the femur, the evidence of a relationship is quite mixed, with the majority of studies showing that volume has no effect on outcome. With the exception of the finding for stomach operations and femur fracture, all the other findings that suggest the lack of a

Table 5.1   Excess deaths in small hospitals

Group & Procedure	Excess deaths	Excess deaths as % of all deaths in small hospitals
Group 1		
Open Heart Surgery	492	38
Vascular Surgery	1327	30
Transurethral resection	396	25
Coronary-artery Bypass	224	41
Group 2		
Colectomy	291	18
Biliary-tract surgery	51	12
Total Hip Replacement	85	43
Resection and Graph, abdominal aortic aneurysm	209	3
Vagotomy and/or pyloroplasty for duodenal ulcer	3	17
Cholecystectomy and incision of common bile duct	4	13
Group 3		
Vagotomy, all	2	27
Cholecystectomy	<1	95

Source: Luft *et al* (1990)

relationship between volume and outcome either have low statistical power; are part of larger analyses in which a physician:volume effect is found; or suggest a causal linkage from outcome to volume. Thus, although a relationship often exists, there is not yet enough evidence to distinguish effects due to physicians from effects due to hospitals or to have much confidence in the relative importance of the causal linkages. (p 177)

The final point leads to a wider one about the link between volume and quality of care: it may work through a number of intermediary variables. Volume, in other words, may reflect factors which tend to be related to hospital size but which are not necessarily linked. For example, bigger hospitals may well have better-trained staff, but staff of similar quality may be found in smaller units. As Flood *et al* (1987) put it:

Volume measures constitute the principal independent measures for explaining differences in quality in the current analyses. However, hospitals as a type of organisation vary along several major structural dimensions that have been found to be associated with quality. Some researchers have found teaching to be associated with better care, particularly for process measure . . . others have found greater expenditures associated with better care and still others have reported evidence that surgery is safer in larger hospitals. Many of the studies did not take multiple structural variables into account at the same time: moreover patient mix often was ignored or was estimated at the hospital level only. Each of these dimensions can, in turn, be expected to be related to volume. (p 297)

The analysis by Flood *et al* did attempt to take on board a large number of structural variables at one and the same time. Their results confirm a volume effect on quality for the surgical categories they used, as well as teaching status and expenditure. However, they also found that larger hospitals did not perform as well as might be expected given their – on average – higher volumes. Furthermore, they found good results where experienced staff worked in smaller, non-teaching hospitals, even though overall, hospital rather than staff variables appeared important and even though volume in each procedure was found to be negatively correlated with mortality. In other words, hospital size as such appeared to have a negative impact on performance. As a consequence, they are cautious about recommending 'regionalisation' if that involved increasing the size of hospitals, as opposed to increasing concentrations of particular types of activity. Their work suggests that benefits from high volume arise in quite narrow ranges of expertise, ie good performance in a particular procedure did not imply good performance in a specialty. This supports Luft *et al*'s argument (1979) that specialisation might best be achieved through medium-sized hospitals concentrating on particular areas of work. However, as these authors recognise, all results must be treated with caution.

In 1995, the newly established NHS Centre for Reviews and Dissemination reviewed the volume/outcome relationship, with particular reference to coronary artery bypass graft surgery, and concluded that:

Whilst most studies report a positive relationship between hospital volume and outcome for several elective procedures, they may have biased estimates of the size of the effect of volume because of poor adjustment for the effect of differences in case-mix between high and low volume hospitals. (p 6)

The research underlying Table 5.1 and a number of other studies assessed in the reviews already cited did recognise that patient characteristics might explain some of the observed relationships and attempted to allow for them by, for example, categorising patients into risk groups or severity categories. But these procedures still leave room for doubt as to their adequacy, which only a randomised trial could dispel.

Moreover, as noted already recognise, many factors influence the quality of care that a hospital offers. Some may be linked to size but not as directly as volume of activity. Thus a study by Shortell and Logerfo (1981) identified a number of factors associated with superior performance including the nature of the links between nurses and other professionals and the extent to which the head of a department was involved in decision-making. Given the small size of their sample, the specific results have to be treated with caution. If they are accepted, the difficult issue is whether their findings relate to hospital scale or scope in any systematic way, or whether they reflect differences in management styles which are not inherent in differences in hospital size.

As the Centre for Reviews and Dissemination (1995) puts it:

> *There is little evidence to show why high volume might be associated with better outcomes and little attempt has been made to 'unpack' this concept. Knowing how well something works is different from knowing how it works. (p 24)*

Thus the precise nature of the links between volume and quality is not perfectly understood. However, the different explanations have different policy implications: for example, if it is the link between the individual clinician and volume that is important, then the quality is 'portable' and volume in the small hospital is irrelevant if the clinical work is done by an itinerant clinician. If the link is with the institutions as a whole, then quality is not portable. Thus in some small hospitals, operations are carried out by surgeons based in larger institutions: if the link is through the individual skill of the clinician, that is a perfectly acceptable form of delivering care. If the link runs through the facilities of the hospital, including the staff supporting the surgeon, as well as the physical equipment, it may not be. Finally, as Flood *et al* point out, if there are quality diseconomies of scale at the level of the hospital, as their analysis suggests, what is right for individual procedures may not be right for all taken together: economies of scale and scope may to some extent conflict.

This is precisely the kind of effect that should be identified or disproved if, for example, the super hospital serving some two million people were to be seriously envisaged. If it were valid for the UK, then it would mean that there might be more complex trade-offs to be examined than were identified in the previous chapter. The benefits of, for example, clustering activities in order to provide the best possible emergency response for the seriously injured might be at the expense of other patients not requiring those facilities.

Furthermore, a statistical connection implies a general relationship not an absolute one. It is perfectly possible for the volume:outcome relationship to be valid, but for some large hospitals to perform badly and some small ones well. The implication is that, before coming to conclusions about the need for change, a means is required of judging the performance of particular units.

The evidence presented so far is virtually all American. However, there is a limited amount of evidence from other sources which bears on the relationship between quality and scale. As shown in Chapter 2, the link between volume and quality may work through the opportunities that larger scale offers to specialisation. The evidence put forward in Chapter 2 suggested that most large hospitals in England are genuinely general institutions. Most retain groupings of general physicians and surgeons, but within those groupings there may nevertheless be considerable specialisation; within general medicine, most hospitals will have specialists in chest, heart and so on. And it is normal for GPs to refer patients to those specialists for outpatient consultations.

However, that does not mean that patients admitted as emergencies will receive specialist care. The management of emergency referrals varies from hospital to hospital, but it is common practice for patients to remain within the control of the 'firm' admitting them who might not contain specialists in their particular condition. Someone referred to an ophthalmologist by a GP will see one, but some who has suffered from a stroke or an asthmatic collapse and is admitted as an emergency may be cared for by a general physician who will of course be familiar with both conditions but who does not consider either a field of special interest.

Dowie's survey (1988) of general medicine found that:

> General medicine is not a specialty that is clearly defined in staffing terms, unlike anaesthetics, for example. Many specialists in fields such as gastroenterology, respiratory diseases or cardiology also accept outpatient referrals of patients with problems of a general nature and they provide care for inpatients who are acutely ill for a variety of medical reasons. Other physicians work solely in their specialised field although, in rheumatology, for example, local practice varies as to whether the consultant is a member of the general acute rota. Local policies differ also over the care of acutely ill elderly patients. Most hospitals have a separate department of medicine for the elderly staffed by consultant geriatricians, but there is no conformity in local admission policies for patients aged 65 years and over ... There are also a few hospitals in which there are not separate departments of general medicine and geriatric

medicine. Rather, consultants have been appointed with responsibility for both the general medical service and the care of the elderly.

Thus patients with similar conditions may be treated in different ways in different parts of the country. In principle, that should have made comparative studies feasible between different hospitals but such studies are rare, and most do not bear on the issues discussed here. However, some studies have been carried out which focus on the relative performance of specialists and generalists. In the case of asthma care, for example, a non-randomised study of 766 admissions in 36 hospitals concluded that respiratory physicians did provide significantly better care than non-respiratory physicians, confirming earlier findings comparing outcomes for patients in general medical units, with and without a specialist respiratory interest (Bucknall *et al*, 1988).

However, the difference was not absolutely clear-cut:

> *Studies from several centres have shown that both the process and outcome of asthma care are significantly better when the teams looking after patients include a respiratory physician ... Such differences should not be surprising; asthma care is central to the work of respiratory physicians who are cognisant of the dangers of acute asthma and familiar with its management and look after many more patients with asthma, including those with more severe asthma, than their colleagues. This survey provides further evidence to demonstrate that there is an advantage in terms of the process of care for those patients looked after by respiratory physicians. Nevertheless, the differences are not absolute and many general physicians continue to provide excellent care. (p 24)*

A recent report on stroke units (Langhorne *et al*, 1991) compared the results of ten studies carried out over the last 30 years. Unlike the volume:outcome studies considered earlier, eight of these used a strict randomisation procedure. All trials involved a specialist multidisciplinary team which provided continuity of care during the first few weeks of illness but they differed in other respects, ie in the precise bundle of interventions provided. Taking the team rather than the individual intervention as the unit of analysis, the authors concluded that there was reliable evidence that specialist units increased chances of reduced mortality. However, they also concluded that:

> *Our overview does not indicate which interventions improve survival. (p 39)*

Although these and other similar studies are not open to the same objections as the volume:outcome work discussed earlier, their interpretation is not straightforward. In some cases, the findings might be ascribed to a 'self-selection' process, ie those operating specialist services may not be representative physicians. While patients may be randomised, it is harder to randomise those treating them. Furthermore, there are risks arising from specialisation – many conditions do not fall clearly within one area or another and particularly older people are likely to suffer from multiple pathology, which a generalist is more likely to identify accurately.

As Jackson (1993) has pointed out:

> *Many surgeons would argue that patients may get a reduced standard of care if they are managed (perhaps unwittingly) by the wrong specialist; that all surgeons know operations sometimes turn out to be very different from expected and especially is this true of emergency operations.*

Thus even if further specialisation would produce better results for the patients directly affected, this would still leave open the question of who deals with patients who do not neatly fall into the interests of one specialty or special service. That risk has been recognised for older people through the emergency of geriatric care as a specialty in its own right, based on a client group where the chances of patients suffering from a number of conditions simultaneously are relatively high and hence the risks of their seeing the 'wrong' specialist all the greater. Furthermore, by nature of their design or the specific areas investigated, the results do not bear on the central issues analysed in Chapters 2 and 3, the advantages to be gained from clustering different but related activities. Thus these findings too must be treated cautiously.

Chapter 3 discussed specialisation between hospitals in the form of hierarchies. As noted there, the case for this form of specialisation can be made in different ways, but ultimately the test is whether the specialist centres at the 'top' of the hierarchy give better results. The Department of Health (1995) published the findings of an expert committee on cancer care which recommended the creation of designated cancer units to deal with the commoner forms of cancer and cancer centres for less common forms. In support of its recommendations, Peter Selby, Professor of Cancer Medicine at the University of Leeds, surveyed the not very extensive literature and concluded as follows:

> *7.1 The literature, supplemented by registry studies, indicates significant improvements in survival as a result of specialist care for a number of cancers both common, moderately*

common and rare. Not all of the studies have been able to adjust adequately for clinical case mix and not all were population based. Numbers are restricted in many studies and not all of the important aspects of patient management have been studied in all studies, presumably because of an inadequate database. This makes it difficult to identify those aspects of specialist care which are most important in each cancer type. These will differ between cancers. For example, colorectal cancer outcomes may be critically dependent on the technical skill of the surgeon; breast cancer outcomes may depend more on the mobilisation of a broad experience of physicians and surgeons.

7.2   *The available literature and Registry data support the case for a specialised cancer service although further work is needed in some cases to define exactly those aspects of such service which are critical for each cancer.*

7.3   *The data suggest that the impact of specialised care for common cancers, and probably for many cancers, can increase long term survival by 5–10%, a very important clinical outcome. (Annex B)*

However, the review noted that 'declared specialists working in district general hospitals . . . were able to produce similar results to declared specialists in colorectal work in teaching hospitals'.

Among the studies cited in Selby's review is one of the management of malignant teratoma (Harding *et al*, 1993), which concluded that centralising treatment did improve outcomes, attributing the advantages of centralisation to both economies of scope and learning by doing:

Thus, our findings and those of previous studies . . . support the contention that it is the cumulative expertise in pathology, radiology, biochemistry, and surgery, in addition to that of the oncology staff, that contributes to the treatment centre survival effect. It is likely that a critical number of patients is needed to develop and maintain this expertise; our data suggest that 10–15 new patients each year may be a reasonable estimate.

This study cannot be considered proof that centralisation of treatment of rare adult tumours improves survival. Although it may be the best evidence currently available, confirmatory data would be welcome. Similar studies in other tumour types are needed to assess the contribution of treatment unit (or surgical team) to outcome to find out whether specialist referral on a large scale can be justified. (p 1002)

These conclusions echo those of the Centre for Reviews and Dissemination; the benefits of specialisation between hospitals remain to be 'unpacked' and the contributions of the various factors which might give rise to them identified separately. Because, within hospitals themselves, there are a large number of care modes even for the same condition, the 'unpacking' process will not be easy. As Kassirer (1994) puts it:

> . . . let us assume that rigorous, reliable, and reproducible methods will be developed to quantify differences between generalists and specialists in the quality of care and that dispassionate researchers are the ones to implement the studies. Such studies could identify which kind of physician is best suited to provide care for acute, life-threatening conditions; whether the outcomes of continuing care for various chronic diseases differ according to the specialty of the physician providing the care; the threshold of clinical severity or complexity at which generalists should refer patients to specialists; and how generalists and specialists should best interact to provide optimal, coordinated care. These data could be the basis for proposals about the number of specialists we need, the proper mix of generalists and specialists, and how the two should work together as a team. We could base decisions, at least in part, on the marginal cost the public is willing to bear for a given marginal benefit. (pp 1151-2)

At present, that marginal benefit cannot be estimated.

Quality and location

So far the evidence, incomplete though it is, tends to point in the same direction, towards concentration as far as some of the main clinical services of the hospital are concerned. However, in Chapter 4, a range of activities were identified which were widely considered appropriate for separation into physically distinct units. Research on quality in such settings is limited: in her review of the small hospital, Higgins (1993) reached the view:

> It has proved difficult to produce genuinely comparable data on outcomes for patients in different settings, including small hospitals, because of the problems of controlling for inputs and patient selection. (p 50)

One reason for this difficulty, apart from the inherent technical issues, is that comparisons between hospitals have been made by enthusiasts for one kind or another. In particular, as Higgins put it:

> small hospital enthusiasts have been assiduous in their attempts to counteract the criticisms and the studies which have been made of clinical outcomes originate with this group. On the basis of the evidence produced to date there are no real reasons to doubt that clinical outcomes in small hospitals can be as good as those in large units if patient selection is carefully monitored and patient throughput is maintained at a reasonable level. However, this

conclusion is drawn on the basis of inadequate data and without the contrary view having been tested fully. (p 51)

In *Community Hospitals: preparing for the future*, the Royal College of General Practitioners (1990) acknowledged that:

At present, there are scanty data on the type of case admitted, the standard of care offered or the outcome of care in Community Hospitals. (p 4)

Nevertheless the reports asserts that:

It is known that the standard of surgery is high, with few complications . . . There is no evidence that centralisation of services in large hospitals improves quality of care . . . .(p 9)

The concluding sentence is clearly overstated in the light of the evidence presented above.

Perhaps the best-analysed service is maternity, in part because many small units still exist. Maternity care is provided in different settings and hence appears to allow comparison of performance, but even here simple comparisons are bedevilled by the difficulty of comparing like cases with like. However, evidence presented to the House of Commons Select Committee on Health (House of Commons, 1992) into maternity care by the National Perinatal Epidemiology Unit at Oxford suggests that:

There is no evidence to support the claim that the safest policy is for all women to give birth in hospital, or the policy of closing small obstetric units on the grounds of safety. (para 26)

The Unit has confirmed this conclusion in the second edition of *Where to be Born* (Campbell and Macfarlane, 1994). It also cites evidence, which the authors themselves do not regard as conclusive, that inpatient care can impose more risks than it avoids.

Here as for other hospital services, one of the keys to separability is patient selection and that in turn depends on the successful application of effective criteria for determining the appropriate place and type of care. The Oxford and the South East Thames strategies and other reports accept that a great deal of elective work is separable into units which do not have the full support systems of a large general hospital. Not all professional opinion accepts that this is safe, even though this is the normal mode of working in the UK private sector and also in many smaller UK hospitals, as well as in free-standing surgi-centres in other countries.

The central question is one of risk. Results reported in the *National Confidential Enquiry into Peri-Operative Deaths (CEPOD)*, both of operations going wrong and of the subsequent transfer, show that a number of the patients were transferred from other hospitals into those where they eventually died, but the precise circumstances of those transfers are not given. The critical question is where the line should be drawn as to what can safely be done in what circumstances, and who should draw it. As things currently stand, decisions are largely left to individual discretion and there is very little by way of systematic evidence to show if that has been abused.

Clearly the extent of the risks will turn on the nature of the procedures carried out. In the case of GP surgery, risks are circumscribed through definition of a list of approved procedure. There is no equivalent for different types of hospital in the UK. A study of minor surgery in GP surgeries and a district general hospital (O' Cathain *et al*, 1992) found that costs were lower in general practice, waiting times shorter, access better in terms of time and cost and satisfaction higher. However, quality was poorer: there were no differences in the rates of wound infection and only one GP patient had subsequently to be referred to a specialist, but GPs incorrectly diagnosed a higher proportion of malignant conditions as benign and inadequately excised 5 per cent of lesions (none in hospital was inadequately excised). As the study concluded, the costs of extra histopathology tests – which GPs were less inclined to use than hospital doctors – which account for their lower detection rate of non-benign conditions – weigh against the health risk from an occasional missed malignancy. The procedures themselves did not appear to pose additional risks in the out-of-hospital environment.

5.2 Service reviews

While medical personnel dominate the acute hospital, the medical profession, at least in the UK, makes few pronouncements on the hospital as a whole bearing on the central issues considered in this report. Individual specialties, on the other hand, frequently do so. But such reports contain very little information – most contain none – which reports on the quality of care currently being delivered. The only regular reporting of hospital performance, the *National Confidential Enquiry into Peri-Operative Deaths,* is carried out under the auspices of the Royal College of Surgeons. Participation in this enquiry is voluntary and hence not all deaths are reported on. But the failings that it has identified are not unlikely to be undermined by that shortfall.

The 1990 report, for example, argued that split site working, where one team of clinicians covers for more than one facility, should be avoided. Its second general recommendation runs:

> *Essential services (including staffed emergency operating rooms, high dependency units and intensive care units) must be provided on a single site wherever emergency/acute surgical care is delivered. (p 11)*

The failings that successive inquiries have identified largely turn on the absence of appropriate expertise and lack of supervision at consultant level, and sometimes of physical facilities. The 1990 report goes on to recommend:

> *Decisions for or against operations should be made jointly by surgeons and anaesthetists: this is a Consultant responsibility. (p 11)*

In general, CEPOD findings support further concentration of services. They do so, however, because it is assumed, realistically enough, that split sites cannot be provided with satisfactory cover of their own and that it is much easier to ensure consultant participation in clinical decision making in larger units. Many accident and emergency facilities continue to be staffed by less experienced personnel and only in a few hospitals are consultants actually on-duty at all times.

A report by the Royal College of Surgeons (1988) also ascribed poor performance, in this case measured by the number of avoidable deaths, to lack of expertise:

> *At present the vast majority of Accident and Emergency Departments in the United Kingdom are supervised by consultants in Accident and Emergency Medicine although most have only one such consultant which is clearly inadequate for a 24 hour day, seven day a week service. (p 10)*

The Royal College report's findings on the quality of care confirmed those of CEPOD, which also found that trauma victims often died because they were seen by inexperienced medical staff without senior colleague involvement. A National Audit Office report (1992)on *Accident and Emergency Departments in England* found that single-handed departments found it hard to guarantee appropriately experienced senior medical cover at all times and that split site working in Worcester, one of the site studies, 'impeded the provision of definitive treatment of severely injured patients'. Other studies have confirmed poor performance: a retrospective study by Anderson and Woodford (1989) found that of 514 patients admitted live to hospital with injuries from which they subsequently died, 20 per cent were judged by four assessors to be preventable and another 13 per cent by three. Another study of the treatment of the management of major trauma (Yates *et al*, 1992) reported on the treatment of seriously injured patients in 33 hospitals: it found that performance (for blunt injuries) was poorer than in comparable US institutions and that there were delays in providing experienced staff to assess and treat patients and in carrying out operations.

The Royal College of Surgeons report on *The Management of Patients with Major Injuries* (1988) also found that there was scope for improvement:

> ... *up to 30 per cent of seriously injured patients who die following admission to the Accident and Emergency Departments of our district general and teaching hospitals do so from potentially treatable causes. Although airway obstruction and insufficiently corrected hypovolaemia are still life threatening hazards one of the main reasons for death is the absence of experienced surgeons able to operate and arrest haemorrhage well within the first hour of admission. Experience suggests that more injured patients die from preventable causes while in hospital than before they reach it. (para 3.3)*

The report contains two analyses of actual performance. The first suggested chances of survival were higher in a (better equipped) teaching hospital; the second, that poor performance was associated with treatment by junior staff.

The Royal College report recommended a two-tier system for dealing with serious injuries, the first being based on the district general hospital, but with 'more consultant involvement' and a second tier through the establishment of a series of trauma centres capable of offering the highest possible standard of care. It proposed, concomitantly, the closure of smaller units now treating serious injuries or, if not closure, a restriction of their work to less threatening conditions, and working in the supervision of a consultant.

A trauma centre has been established at Stoke to test out the ideas set out in this report. So far, however, no information is available as to how the Centre compares with conventional accident and emergency departments. A number of evaluations of trauma centres have been published in the US, but because the hospital systems of the two countries are different, it is hazardous to transfer the results. However, here too a volume effect has been identified. To take one example, a study by Smith *et al* (1990) found a significant relationship between the volume of seriously injured patients seen and survival rates at each trauma centre.

Again, however, the volume effect has to be 'unpacked'. Better performance may be due to better equipment, access to associated specialties, effective management with A&E departments and, above all, to the skills and availability of medical staff.

The British Association for Accident and Emergency Medicine (1993) attributed poor performance in UK hospitals to inappropriate staffing and hence proposed on-site senior/middle grade presence for at least 16 hours a day, seven days a week, with full consultant cover on call. Their report recognises that smaller centres would find it hard to provide this level of cover and it therefore recognises the trade-off between quality and access, suggesting that in sparse rural areas, purchasers may decide to provide a similar standard of service to elsewhere, accepting the higher cost of that as the price of accessibility. A study carried out in Northern Ireland suggested that this approach could produce good quality care; in that study (McNicholl *et al*, 1993) the level of preventable deaths was fairly low, varying between 4 and 15 per cent, but no significant difference was found between large and small hospitals in saving those who could be saved. However, there was a high level of consultant involvement, particularly in the smaller hospitals. On that basis, the authors concluded that there was no case for the centralisation of emergency care into trauma centres in the area studied. No cost data were presented.

The significance of this study, however, is not straightforward. While it does support the view that size as such is not important, it is not sufficient to disprove the case for concentration on to a smaller number of sites. If good outcomes are associated with experienced staff making quicker and more accurate diagnoses or carrying out procedures more efficiently, then the best policy could be to ensure that expertise was used to its maximum effect. Within accident and emergency services and the related specialties of trauma and orthopaedics, the case for concentrating the most skilled staff arises in part from the requirements of offering a 24-hour service and the advantages of a larger workforce from which to draw to do so. If staff of a particular sort is limited in number in the short to medium term, it may be best to deploy it where it can be used to best advantage. In the short and medium term, it is generally assumed that experienced medical manpower in the UK is nearly in fixed supply. If that is so, then the critical question is not: do large units do better than small ones, but do the available medical resources work more effectively in larger units?

5.3 Conclusion

Overall, the evidence suggests links of several kinds between volume and outcome may exist, but it is impossible to determine from the sources cited here and the studies they review, the relative importance of each determining factor. Nevertheless, unless the observed relationships arise entirely because of the characteristics of patients, ie if larger hospitals or busier surgeons were treating more physically fit patients, then concentration should provide benefits in terms of reduced mortality since concentration backs all strands of the volume:outcome hypothesis, provided it does not take hospitals as a whole past their point where quality falls.

But a volume:outcome relationship, even if demonstrated, is only one element in a broader picture. A large number of questions remain which only systematic analysis of clinical performance in different settings can resolve: the precise division of the role between institutions, the desirable scale of particular units and the implications, if some work becomes very highly concentrated, for related clinical activities for which the same results are not available. The framework for analysis set out in Chapters 2 to 4 emphasised the importance of linkages between the various activities carried out in a general hospital; but most of the studies cited here, or in the reviews this chapter has drawn on, consider only one small area of activity at a time.

Furthermore, the planning and implementation of change are disruptive, so it is important to know in advance what the potential scale of benefits might be. That question has been answered for the US for a number of common procedures in terms of the number of deaths which would be averted by a regionalisation (ie concentration) programme covering several hundred hospitals, assuming that the observed differences between small and large hospitals were real.

Using data for 1972, Maerki *et al* (1986) derived estimates of 'potentially averted deaths' shown in the first column in Table 5.2, similar to those in Table 5.1. The second column relates these to the number of patients whose care would have to be shifted to realise this potential. The ratio varies widely from over 1 in 10 to one in 1,000. As the authors point out, even if these results are valid, other factors must be taken into account, principally, in line with the analysis presented here, issues of cost and access.

> *While policy decisions concerning regionalisation must incorporate a wide range of factors, the disruption implicit in regionalisation may offset the anticipated benefits. For example we should ask whether we want to transfer 11,255 cirrhosis patients to reduce the number of deaths from 1,571 to 1,530. Might it not be better to transfer 18,000 patients requiring a total hip replacement to reduce the number of deaths from 910 to 313? (p 157)*

Table 5.2   Total potentially averted deaths (averted deaths per 1,000 patients shifted)

Fracture of femur	4.5
Peptic ulcer	1
Acute MI	20
Stomach operations	8
Hysterectomy	1
Abdominal aortic aneurysm	107
Intestinal operations	16
Cholecystectomy	2
Cardiac catheterization	14
Cardiac bypass	37
Transurethral prostatectomy	1
Hernia repair	0.5
Respiratory distress syndrome	17
Cirrhosis	4
Appendectomy	1
Total hip replacement	32

Source: Maerki *et al* (1986)

The authors go on to stress the complexities once the total picture is taken into account.

> *There are marked differences across types of conditions in the life-saving potential of regionalisation efforts. To investigate further specific policy alternatives, one should know the travel times and transportation costs both monetary and medical, associated with regionalisation. If the low-volume hospitals are geographically close to high volume hospitals with good outcomes then such costs may be small, but important referral patterns may have to be altered. If lower-volume hospitals with poor outcomes are in isolated areas, greater care must be taken in recommending regionalisation (p 157).*

It is not possible to make similar estimates for the UK from readily available information. At a national level, no data are regularly published on the volume of activity within each hospital. However, the data made available by the National Case Mix Office to the King's Fund can be used to indicate the extent to which procedures and treatments are concentrated in a small number of providers, or the reverse.

The evidence presented in Chapter 2 suggested that general hospitals in England are indeed general. The same source of data can be used to show, for a narrow range of procedures and diagnoses, chosen because most of the US research studies applies to them, what the present pattern of activity is. In the case of heart transplant surgery, there has been a national policy to limit the number of centres carrying out this form of work. Consequently, levels of activity are high in nearly all the identified providers.

The same is not true for the other procedures and diagnoses. Table 5.3 presents information on the frequency with which a number of procedures are carried out where the evidence for a scale effect is relatively strong. In all cases, a large number of units are found to be working at very low levels of activity.

Table 5.3 Volume of activity: selected procedures: England 1991/92

	No. of providers carrying out less than 10 procedures per year
Procedures/diagnosis	
Cholecystectomy	32
Transurethral resection of prostate	25
Inguinal hernia repair	21
Hysterectomy	27
Appendectomy	30
Fracture of neck of femur	106
Acute myocardial infarction	100
CABG	10
Abdominal aortic aneurysm	96
Total hip replacement	33

Source: King's Fund Policy Institute analysis

As already emphasised, these data refer to provider units and not individual surgeons or physicians: to an unknown degree some of the 'tail' of small-scale provision might be carried out by experienced staff working away from their main hospital. Because of the confidentiality restrictions within which these data were obtained, the individual provider units cannot be identified. Even if this could be done, as they stand the data are not guides to action, but they are guides to questions which purchasers might raise about performance in those units handling very low volumes. Although, in the light of the previous discussion, any conclusions about volume effects must be qualified, nearly all the evidence cited in this chapter and the material they in turn call on support the view that very low levels of activity are to be avoided.

Furthermore, in some circumstances, particularly accident and emergency departments, it appears that poor performance is due to factors not inherently linked to scale of activity such as the expertise of those providing the service. If so, then the critical questions turn on the link between the volume of activity and the acquisition and maintenance of that expertise, and also on the way that experienced staff are deployed, ie whether they are part of the 'front-line' service or act primarily as medical managers, and on the scope allowed inexperienced staff to work unsupervised. Overall, therefore, it is hard to dissent from the conclusion reached by the NHS Centre for Reviews and Dissemination:

> ... policy-makers should be cautious when invoking the assumed improvements in outcome achieved by volume as a key argument for centralisation of service

However, our reservations stem not only from the methodological qualifications set out in the Centre's Report, but also from the framework for analysis set out in Chapters 2 and 3. In particular, if the links between specialties are important, examination of each one in isolation risks ignoring significant inter-actions between them.

CHAPTER 6

Scale, scope and costs

Although costs of provision may seem to pose relatively straightforward issues in comparison with clinical quality, it proves just as hard to find evidence of the kind required by the framework set out in the previous part. That framework requires an understanding of how costs of provision change as a result of changes in hospital configuration. At its simplest, it means identifying whether units which do more work of a given kind have lower costs per case than units which do less, ie whether there is a volume/cost relationship. But while it is important to establish whether this is or is not the case, it represents only a fraction of what ideally we need to know.

The main conclusion drawn earlier was that the large range of services on which hospitals rely could not be assumed to exhibit the same relationships between activity level and costs. If that is correct, then an understanding of the key relationships would have to be based on a series of individual studies of particular aspects of hospital activity; the basic unit of analysis might be the speciality or the individual support function. The volume:cost relationship at the level of the hospital as a whole sheds little light on how costs vary for particular services, but as most of the evidence is of the former sort, it is that which must be considered, taking first scale and then scope.

6.1 Scale

Most studies of hospital costs have taken a macro or global approach, looking at hospital activity as a whole and hence grouping together literally thousands of different activities. A large number of such studies have been carried out, mainly in the US, which have attempted to establish whether or not costs vary with size. In the vast majority of cases, this work has been carried out without consideration of outcomes, ie it has focused on cost per case or per patient day.

When allowances are made for patient characteristics, particularly age and diagnosis, scale effects are not usually found to be large and, where they exist, apply over only a limited range. During the 1970s, the Department of Health's Operational Research Service found that revenue costs per case rose, often allowing for specialty (but not case) mix above 370 beds, at that time a fairly low level for a general hospital. The Department of Health Estates Directorate, using data from the 1980s to identify the advantages of different designs of hospital, found no scale effects: there were wide differences in costs, measured as cost per case, at all size levels. This study also failed fully to take into account case-mix.

More recently, using data from the 1990s, Bartlett and Le Grand (1993) found, in a study of hospitals in England, that ward costs rose with increasing scale. Ward costs form a little over half of hospital costs and include the bulk of nursing expenditure, but they do not take into account support costs, including services such as heating and catering which might for technical reasons be subject to increasing returns to scale. Furthermore, the authors were not able to allow for differences in case-mix. If, as might be expected, the larger hospitals handle the more seriously injured or seriously ill and complex categories of work, then some increase in costs per case is only to be expected. Evans (1971) pointed out in a study of Canadian hospitals that, although it appeared that hospitals with over 1,000 beds had higher costs, this effect might be due to differential case severity. The same author concluded (1972) that the pattern of discharge diagnoses is this crucial determinant of inter-hospital variations in cost per case and per day:

There is very little evidence of impact on costs from scale of plant once diagnostic and age-sex mix and other sorts of activities are adjusted for. (p 417)

Furthermore, it may be that the demand facing larger hospitals is more variable than that facing small ones and hence a greater level of spare capacity is required for any given level of confidence that demand can be met.

These points serve to underline how difficult it is to measure the relationship between costs and hospital activity, even at a global level. What evidence there is suggests that the existence of scale economies cannot be taken for granted as they would be in most production industries. Given the nature of hospital costs, this result is not surprising. As Table 6.1 shows, the bulk of hospital costs lie in nursing. As the scale of a hospital increases, essentially further units of nursing service, as well as other bed, patient and ward-related costs are added, such as domestic and catering expenditure. The nature of what is done is more or less the same.

But it would be wrong to infer from the apparent weakness of the scale effect that existing hospitals could be split up into their component functions with no consequences for costs.

Table 6.1   Hospital cost structures

		%
Patient treatment	68.6	
Wards		53.2
Outpatients		5.7
A&E		2.8
Community nursing/midwifery		8.7
Operating theatres		7.2
Pathology		5.3
Radiology		4.0
Other departments		13.2
General	31.4	
Domestic		8.6
Catering		10.6
Engineering maintenance		8.1
Building maintenance		5.9
Water & sewage		6.8
Site overheads		20.9
Office support		14.6
Training & education		6.8
Other		17.9

Source: Welsh Health Costing Returns

Obviously, existing institutions embody a large amount of fixed capital which cannot readily be redeployed into other uses. Practical experience of the impact of reducing the scale of existing hospitals suggests that it is difficult to reduce costs pro rata when bed capacity is reduced (Beech and Larkinson, 1990).

However, that results in part from the existence of costs which are contractually fixed in the short and medium term, such as personnel on long term contracts, as well as fixed capital costs which cannot be quickly reduced. Over time, the fixed becomes the variable as capital can be withdrawn and put to other uses and staff redeployed. Nevertheless, indivisibilities will remain, which are dictated by technical factors such as the minimum size for a CT scanner and, as suggested in Chapter 2, some functions such as heating and other support services will be subject to scale economies for technical reasons.

Although it seems reasonable to assume that there are cost thresholds throughout the whole range of hospital services, there is no reason nor evidence to suggest they occur at the same points. Indeed, the apparent absence of economies of scale at overall hospital level in itself suggests they do not. Thus at any given hospital size, some services are likely to be operating at their most efficient point, some will have spare capacity and others are being used more intensively than is economic. In the latter case, the extra costs may, however, be reflected in delays to patients and other aspects of quality rather than in the costs of the hospital itself: for example, if capacity is used too intensively, the ability of the hospital to cope with variations in demand is reduced. In this case unit costs may fall, along with quality. Bartlett and Le Grand found, for example, that for any given size of hospital unit costs fell with utilisation. This is exactly what one expects in any organisation with some degree of fixed costs and a level of capacity set to meet a variable demand.

Where there are cost thresholds, then low costs will turn primarily on matching workload to capacity. That is one reason why, where demand is variable, the large unit has an inherent advantage over the small since in proportionate terms its need for spare capacity is less. That possible source of advantage was noted in Chapter 2; however, the documents cited there do not present any figures for the cost savings which might result from 'pooling' capacity.

In contrast, small or medium-sized hospitals may in some circumstances be able to match capacity to demand as well as large, and produce low cost care. But that does not mean that such units are efficient taken the overall workload of hospitals. For example, a separate elective unit could, by planning its workload, operate at a very high level of utilisation, and provide care at a lower cost than one situated in a general hospital taking emergency cases as and when required to. However, it may be more efficient, taking elective and emergency together, to run the two types of service with the same bedstock as do the vast majority of British hospitals, at least as far as hospital costs alone are concerned. If costs of cancellation and delay to patients were included, the balance of advantage might be different; there appears to be no empirical evidence on the scale of these costs.

A further limitation of the work cited so far is that it looks at the situation at a point in time, rather than over a period of time. The workload of hospitals is constantly changing as are the methods used to cope with it. If practice makes perfect, then both cost as well as quality should improve with time or experience. Evidence of the existence of this effect on costs comes from a number of studies relating to particular procedures.

A study of heart transplantation in Indiana (Woods *et al*, 1992) followed the cost of treating patients over a four year period. The costs per patient fell rapidly during this period but the volume per year did not rise so, the authors suggest, there was no volume effect as such. The model fitted to the data suggests that the fiftieth case would be 31 per cent of the cost of the first.

Studies by Munoz *et al* (1990a-d) on a range of surgical procedures have found similar results. In the case of neurosurgery, the authors found that there were sharp cost distinctions between low and high volume surgeons though outcomes did not differ: see Table 6.2. The higher volume surgeons kept their patients in hospital for fewer days and the costs of carrying out the procedures nearly $2,000 less. In respect of oncology, the same authors found both a cost and quality (mortality) relationship with volume.

Table 6.2 Length of stay and cost per case and physician volume for non-emergency neurosurgical patients

Category	Low-volume neurosurgeons	High-volume neurosurgeons
Sample size	145	630
Patients per physician	1.6	45
Hospital length of stay (days)	6.88 ± 8.60	4.43 ± 4.18
Total hospital cost ($)	5,865 ± 6,880	4,070 ± 3,655

Source: Munoz *et al* (1990a)

As the authors recognise, however, these findings are subject to the same qualification as those attached to studies of volume and outcomes, the mix of patients for the two groups of surgeons may not have been identical.

In this country, a study by Opit *et al* (1991) found that more experienced staff took less operating theatre time. They estimated that cost would be lower by 11.3 per cent if all operations in the areas cited were carried out by the most experienced staff.

The impact of learning on costs should of course affect all hospitals and so might be irrelevant to the central issues of this report unless it was only in larger units that the necessary experience could be gained and deployed. If the volume/cost effect works through the individual clinician, moving individuals around should allow the value of experience to be enjoyed in different settings, no matter where it is gained.

The apparent link between experience and cost levels suggest that if the 'collegiate' arguments for concentration are valid, then this should show itself in better cost as well as quality performance. Whether it does or not, it is not possible to say: costs are higher in the main centres of teaching and research when measured on a cost per case basis, but this is usually attributed to the costs of providing for teaching or the higher than average complexity of cases. Some work (Garber *et al*, 1984) suggests that even when these are accounted for, costs in teaching establishments are higher – though quality might be higher as well.

Part of the case for clustering activities turns on the possibility that they create scale advantage in support services. In Chapter 2, it was pointed out that contracting out may allow economies of scale to be enjoyed by small as well as large institutions. Stilwell (1993) argues that the configuration of pathology services can be largely independent of the size of the hospital because the way that these services are supplied can be adapted to the circumstances of the hospital. As his analysis shows, complete physical and managerial separation from other hospital functions is feasible for most diagnostic functions normally included in pathology services. Hence small and large hospitals should be able to enjoy similar cost levels. The same appears to be true for other support services through the availability of contracting out; however, in some, more rural, parts of the country, effective markets may not exist and hence hospitals may be forced to provide in-house (Milne, 1993).

6.2 Scope

In most studies of hospital costs, no distinction is made between scale and scope, ie size of hospital has been measured in terms such as bedstock or caseload which does not distinguish the range of work done. But a few studies have recognised that hospitals are 'multi-product' firms and hence that a distinction between the two must be maintained. Some have identified the existence of scope economies: for example a micro study (Hillson *et al*, 1992) looked in detail at the work of doctors within hospitals, estimating the cost and time of providing a number of common services in isolation or together. They found that 'work savings associated with providing services together ranged from 4 to 30 per cent of the total work of the separate services.' However, the areas of work considered were small relative to the total work of the hospital so the results do not bear on the interactions between clinical specialties that were suggested above as being central to the case for clustering. Another micro study (Dunn *et al*, 1995) identified economies of scope in the performance of multiple surgery, but this again comprises a small part of total hospital activity.

A different result was obtained by Granneman *et al* (1986), who found that hospitals with larger inpatient volumes had higher costs in their emergency departments. How might this be explained? As they suggest:

> *One possibility is that the larger range of services offered and the greater difficulty of co-ordinating diverse hospital activities account for this result. It could also be the case that large hospitals have emergency department visits that are more complex (or costly) in ways not captured by our case-mix measures. Alternatively, having a large emergency department may increase the average complexity of admissions, given case-mix. (p 122)*

The latter explanation seems a likely one since it seems plausible that the larger departments will attract the more difficult cases, in which case this study does not demonstrate diseconomies of scope. The same study found economies of scale within emergency departments but not in outpatients. That finding is in line with what one might expect from points set out earlier. The emergency department is subject to variable demand, and hence should enjoy scale economies: outpatients are planned, labour-intensive functions, which are less likely to.

Carr and Feldstein (1967) looked at scope and scale together: scope was measured by what they termed service capability groups. They found that the larger the number of groups a hospital provided, the larger the hospital had to be to attain low cost levels in each. Diseconomies of scale were observed only in the hospital active in all groups. Thus the analysis suggested that small hospitals with wide scope would be high cost, while large hospitals with narrow scope would not offer cost advantages to offset higher access costs.

A more recent study by Cowing and Holtmann (1983) suggested a different conclusion: that while some economies of scope could be identified, these appeared to be outweighed by diseconomies:

> *These results also have significant policy implications, especially since the current policy of merging smaller hospitals into larger institutions providing a full array of services is implicitly grounded upon the premise of economies of scope, i.e., cost savings from joint production. Our results suggest that such policies may be misplaced and that the unconditional consolidation of existing hospital services may not generally be appropriate on strict efficiency grounds. Thus, it would appear that any potential cost savings from joint production can be realized only through the selective merging of some hospital services, and that caution should be exercised in selecting those particular services to be combined. In general, our results on both scope and scale effects indicate that large but more (rather than less) specialized hospitals may be more*

cost-effective, given the significance of our estimated scale effects and the general lack of any substantial economies of scope. (p 650)

On this evidence, it appeared better to have larger specialised hospitals in order to enjoy scale economies within any one service without countervailing increases in costs overall.

These studies, with their contrasting results, carried out with a much larger quantity of data than is available in the UK, serve to underline the remarks at the beginning of this chapter. No UK studies directly address the issue of scope, but some bear on it indirectly, by considering the implications of carrying out particular work in different settings, specifically large general hospitals and smaller units. If economies of scope or scale existed, then the expectation would be that the smaller units would show higher costs. But if the two kinds of hospitals are acting primarily as complements, at different ends of the overall hospital market, the expectation would be that average costs would differ. Whether overall it would cost more or less to shift activity one way or the other cannot be answered by studies of this kind.

Furthermore, a drawback of the work cited and similar studies is that they focus on hospitals as they are, whereas recent proposals for the development of hospitals imply the creation of institutions of a type which do not presently exist at least in the UK, such as major free-standing surgical facilities, or of which there is as yet little experience, such as the local hospital carrying out the range of functions set out in Chapter 3. Moreover, in order to understand the economic consequences of reconfiguring services, the impact of detaching some functions in whole or part from the existing cluster of activities and putting them in alternative clusters must be estimated. This is particularly critical if there are economies of scope. In these circumstances, withdrawal of some services from the 'main' hospital may undermine the economics of the whole.

In other sectors, the standard approach to dealing with issues of this kind is to build up 'theoretical' costs, either by statistical inference or 'engineering' studies or other modelling methods. There is very little work of this kind for the hospital as a whole or its separate functions. However, detailed studies of nursing costs by Stilwell and Hawley (1991) indicate the importance of looking at the way costs vary at a very detailed level. They found that nursing costs varied a great deal in apparently similar circumstances and were some-times very low as some patients made very few demands on nursing resources. They conclude:

One of the most important lessons of the wide range of observed costs is that although some patients are expensive in nursing terms, many are extremely cheap.

Our methodology entails at least an average charge to cover the cost of activities such as housekeeping, but even so, a quarter of patients cost less than £13 a day in total. Keeping a patient in an acute hospital for particular tests, recuperation or social reasons need not, therefore, always be as expensive and implicitly wasteful as is usually represented. (p 3)

On this basis, savings from reduced length of stay or accelerated discharge may be very small indeed, or even negative, if only low cost patients were discharged early. They may be much larger if as a result of shorter stays, other changes can be made which allow costs elsewhere to be reduced, ie if overall throughput could be increased, capital and other costs might be saved.

6.3 Conclusion

Taking what evidence does exist, it would seem that neither scale nor scope appears to confer large cost advantages (Cowing *et al*, 1983). While this suggests that small can compete with large in terms of costs, it does not bear on the implications of a more thorough-going dispersal away from hospitals as they are now into a wide range of settings. Here the individual thresholds become critical. If, for example, expensive diagnostic equipment were sited 'in the community', it could only operate as efficiently as within a hospital if the same volume of use could be created.

Overall, the evidence presented in this chapter is patchy and what exists is subject to similar methodological limitations to that presented in the previous chapter. These arise from differences in severity within a category of care, differences in the mix of categories and in the complexity of the underlying cost relationships. To a large degree, that reflects the difficulties outlined earlier of relating costs in a useful way to what hospitals do, ie the case-mix and variations in severity within case-mix categories. It also reflects a lack, particularly in the UK, of usable data at the hospital level and of the poor quality of hospital costing systems. A study of hospital costs in Australia (Butler, 1995) concluded:

One may well speculate . . . whether there would be greater returns from the production of more relevant data than from the application of more econometrics to existing types of data. (p 361).

Given the meagre results presented here, it is hard to disagree with that conclusion. In particular circumstances, the cost implications of locational substitution of post-operative nursing care may perhaps be best estimated when the implications of specific reconfigurations of services are being considered. Even for this purpose, however, better costing systems than those which currently exist are required.

But for other purposes, more than this is required. The question raised by Kassirer (1994), cited in Chapter 5, of how the marginal benefit of extra specialisation relates to the marginal cost of producing it, cannot be answered by looking at hospital costs alone, at a given point in time. Rather, it involves an examination of the overall process by which different degrees of specialisation are achieved, as well as the actual deployment of that expertise. That would require detailed cost evidence over substantial periods of time, and of a type not considered in any of the studies cited in this chapter.

CHAPTER 7

Access

Within the framework developed in Chapter 2, the central question posed by access costs is how they should be 'traded-off' against the advantages, in terms of quality and cost, that clustering and concentration of activities may produce. For some patients, clustering can yield accessibility benefits since in any one visit, they may make use of a range of specialist facilities. For the most part, however, it seems reasonable to assume that fewer sites for the delivery of hospital services would mean longer and more expensive trips.

The analysis suggested that access costs fell into three categories:

- costs to the NHS of providing ambulance and car services
- travel costs incurred by patients/relatives and visitors
- clinical costs, incurred by the time and discomfort of travel to hospital or by any reduction in utilisation which access costs in the wide sense may impose.

This chapter attempts to identify the significance of each of these for the structure of hospital provision.

7.1 Financial costs

Overall, ambulance services costs some £400m per year, a small fraction of the total hospitals budget. Not surprisingly, there is a wide variation in cost per head in different areas, with rural areas showing the highest figures. In Wales, with both heavily urbanised and deeply rural areas, costs range from £4 to £19 per head of population and £10 to £46 per trip: see Tables 7.1 and 7.2.

According to the National Audit Office (1990), whereas 40 years ago ambulance services carried only emergency cases, now over 85 per cent are non-emergencies. The vast majority of ambulance service costs fall on the NHS: only NHS patients who are medically unfit to travel by other means are entitled to use of ambulances: low income is not a relevant criterion.

Table 7.1   Welsh ambulance services 1988-89: cost per head of population

	£
Powys	19
Gwynedd	15
East Dyfed	10
Gwent	9
Mid Glamorgan	8
Pembrokeshire	8
Clwyd	8
South Glamorgan	8
West Glamorgan	7
Great Britain	6

Source: National Audit Office (1990)

Table 7.2   Welsh ambulance services 1988-89: non-emergency patient journeys per 1,000 population

Powys	720
Gwent	630
Mid Glamorgan	520
West Glamorgan	500
Pembrokeshire	500
South Glamorgan	480
Gwynedd	400
Clwyd	360
East Dyfed	330
Great Britain	350

Source: National Audit Office (1990)

What counts as medical need is subject to different interpretations and as a result, in the words of the report:

> *a more flexible interpretation of medical need may be applied to patients without access to public or private transport. (p 12)*

Some ambulance services charge patients where medical need is not established, but this is not an established pattern.

The limited role of NHS provision reflects the underlying policy that responsibility for getting to hospital, except in narrowly defined circumstances, falls to the patient. There has been no commitment, matching that in the provision of hospital services themselves, to ensuring (rough) equality of access.

Although the overall cost of ambulance services is low relative to NHS costs as a whole, they may nevertheless form a significant part of the costs of changing the disposition of hospital emergency care because mileage costs are already high and likely to get higher as the skill levels of ambulance crews is raised.

The significance of access costs is, however, increased when the access costs falling on patients are taken into account. There are no comprehensive data relating to travel to hospitals and where the burden of financing them lies. The National Travel Surveys, carried out for the Department of Transport, give information on the number of trips made to health facilities including hospitals, and the mode of travel used. The Survey does not always distinguish hospitals from GP surgeries and other health facilities, but it nevertheless does shed some light on access issues. Table 7.3 shows travel to health facilities by age and mode, using data from the most recent survey.

Table 7.3 Mode of access to health facilities

Age	Walk	Car	Public transport
All	10.3	65.8	17.1
65–69	10.3	59.8	21.5
85+	16.3	48.9	28.0

Source: National Travel Survey, 1989-91

About two thirds of trips to hospital are made by car, and for most, the distances to be covered are not very great, but the proportion falls sharply with age and is less than half for the very elderly, over a quarter of whom use public transport.

The Survey does not give actual journey times, but a number of small-scale studies carried out in particular parts of the country have examined them. These reveal that, for some people, travel to hospital is both time-consuming and expensive and sometimes very difficult. Certain groups of the population find journeys to hospital arduous and expensive, particularly elderly people, mothers with children and those with disabilities that make some forms of transport hard to use.

Pearson (1992) surveyed over 300 people in low income areas of Merseyside: 78 of them were interviewed. Her work identified a number of people who could not get to outpatient appointments, particularly early morning ones, without 'borrowing' time from others. In other words, complicated re-arrangements of domestic regimes and arrangements with family, friends and neighbours were required which were not always easy to achieve. A similar conclusion emerged from a survey by the Welsh Consumer Council (1988) of access to outpatient clinics:

> *Time was a more pressing consideration for mothers and child-escorts than for the elderly. They were more likely to have to get home by a certain time to see to children and many were anxious or worried during their visit to the clinic about when they would get home. More than a third did not know whether they might be entitled to hospital transport.*
>
> *Child-escorts reported greatest difficulty travelling by bus and many complained about the absence of a direct service. Two out of five lost pay as a result of bringing their child to the clinic. (p 5)*

A study in Northern Ireland by Reid and Todd (1989) identified long journey times to a rural outpatient clinic; of those using public transport or walking, over half had a round trip in excess of an hour and 15 per cent had a round trip of over two hours. Most of these patients did not have access to a car and the bus service did not directly link the bus terminal and the rail station with the hospital. Not surprisingly, they found a considerable demand for a direct bus service.

The conclusion which emerges from the evidence cited here is straightforward and in line with what one would expect. For most people, most of the time, access to hospital services is not difficult, but it can be for some groups, depending on their economic and social circumstances, as well as their location.

Nevertheless, even if people are able to make trips to hospitals easily enough and are not deterred from using them by distance, they still have to incur costs in doing so. For some, the critical costs may not be the journey itself, but the 'opportunities lost' in making it. Cartwright and Windsor (1992) found in a study of outpatient attendances that the total impact could be considerable taking into account loss of working time: the average time lost was over two days and a few lost a week or more: see Table 7.4.

Table 7.4 Working time lost due to patients' attendance at hospital

	%
Less than I hour	7
I hour < 3 hours	18
3 hours < 6 hours	28
6 hours < I day	8
I day < 2 days	11
2 days < 3 days	7
3 days < I week	5
I week or more	16
Number of patients in work (= 100%)	162
Average time lost	2 days 5 hours

Source: Cartwright and Windsor (1992)

Unlike ambulance costs, access and opportunity costs fall on patients and there is no compensation for them. As a result, the choice between access, cost and quality is distorted since health care providers and purchasers do not have to meet all the costs on both sides of the equation. Not surprisingly therefore, attempts to relate travel costs incurred by patients and visitors to costs incurred within the hospital are rare. Nevertheless some have been made.

In the late 1970s, detailed studies were carried out in the Bath and Oxford areas of the travel costs incurred in attending paediatrics clinics in different locations (Cullis *et al*. 1981). These calculated the value of the time spent travelling as well as the monetary costs of travel, drawing on the methods used by the Department of Transport to value time in the appraisal of transport projects. These attach a value both to time lost from working hours and also – at a lower rate – non-working time.

The central clinic was cheaper for the NHS: £787 as opposed to £634 per 100 cases. But if travel and time costs were taken into account, the balance of advantage was changed: the central clinics were estimated to cost in total £688 more than the peripheral ones: see Table 7.5.

On this basis, taking the costs to users into account alongside NHS costs would have led to a different choice. The same conclusion emerged from a study of operations in different hospitals in the same district. Soper and Jones (1985) found, using Department of Transport values of time, that differences in travel costs made a decisive contribution to changing the ranking of the options they considered: Option Q – centralisation in DGHs – was found to be the most expensive by virtue of the £141,000 additional travel costs; Option S – which involved

Table 7.5 Comparison of typical central and peripheral outpatient sessions for a cohort of 100 attendances

Cost, benefit type	Peripheral patients at Oxford clinics (1)	Peripheral patients at peripheral clinics (2)	Differences (1) - (2) (3)
Direct Tangible Benefits			
a) Car costs	£332.83	£ 51.03	£281.80
b) Public transport fares	£ 16.42	£ 4.92	£ 11.50
c) Ambulance costs (an internal cost)	£ 77.09	£ 12.40	£ 64.69
d) Special expenses	£ 17.82	£ 0.59	£ 17.23
Indirect Tangible Benefits			
e) Lost market production (fathers)	£422.35	£149.58	£272.77
f) Lost market production (mothers)	£ 95.88	£ 26.97	£ 68.91
Indirect Tangible Benefits			
g) Lost non-market production (fathers)	£ 24.74	£ 12.13	£ 12.61
h) Lost non-market production (mothers)	£ 71.39	£ 44.79	£ 26.60
I) Lost non-market production (children)	£180.70	£ 96.04	£ 84.66
j) Net unit internal cost of 100 POPC (but also see row c)	£634.00	£787.00	-£153.00
k) Net differential in overall: money sum [(a) to (j)]	£687.77		
l) Internal costs as % overall money sum: [(j) + (c)] divided by [(a) to (j)] × 100	37.96%	67.43%	

Source: Cullis *et al* (1981)

Table 7.6   Capital and social costs and changes in revenue costs of four options (£000)

Options	Number of theatres	Patients travelling	Equivalent annual capital costs	Annual revenue costs	Social costs
Local hospitals					
P	4	603	192	0	26
Q	0	0	0	0	0
R	2	349	96	0	13
S	3	1050	144	-14	41
District general hospitals					
P	0	0	0	0	0
Q	3	3474	144	-19	141
R	1	982	48	-14	49
S	0	0	0	0	0

Option	Total cost change
P	218
Q	266
R	192
S	171

Source: Soper and Jones (1985)

investing in theatres in local hospitals – proved to be the cheapest, taking all costs into account: see Table 7.6.

These examples suggest that concentration on NHS costs alone would bias choices in favour of centralisation of facilities. How the costs falling on users should be estimated is not straightforward but established conventions of time and operating costs are in use for other public sector decisions and so might reasonably be applied to the provision of health services.

7.2 Clinical costs

The general expectation for all kinds of travel is that distance reduces the number of trips made to any type of destination. However, given the importance of trips to hospital, this effect may be expected to be relatively modest – much less for example than trips made to leisure facilities which can be regarded as optional. In other words, the time and cost of trips may not influence the number made, except perhaps for visitors, whose trips may also be said to be optional.

Where, as in metropolitan areas, there are alternative facilities, access costs and more specifically times appear to be important determinants of use of particular hospitals. However, according to one study of an area containing a number of hospitals (McGurk and Porell, 1984), their importance as influences on behaviour appears to vary between services: surgical patients were found to be more sensitive to time and cost differences than gynaecological patients.

However, this study looked at choice of hospital rather than total hospital use. Here we find a different pattern. Roos and Lyttle (1985) studied the consequences of centralising total hip replacement in Manitoba, a large and sparsely settled province of Canada, and concluded that differential access had had no impact on access as between residents of the urban centres where surgery was centralised and other residents of the province. Similarly, Carstairs and Morris (1991) found in Scotland that there was little difference in rates of hospital use as between urban and rural areas. More surprising, it appeared that deprivation did not appear to reduce use of hospital. However, that might hide a greater than average need for service.

Haynes and Bentham's study (1979) found contradictory evidence as far as hospital inpatient stays were concerned. Although people reported they were deterred, analysis of the 'objective' information about hospital episodes suggested that people in the remoter rural areas were not under-using hospital facilities relative to better located groups. However, in a later study (Haynes and Bentham, 1982) a significant impact on attendance at outpatient clinics was observed among non-car owners and also non-manual workers: there were similar differences in the other groups identified but not a statistically significant level: see Table 7.7. Consultation rates were lower in rural areas for all the groups identified; the same is true of outpatients.

The obvious interpretation of these findings is that demand for inpatient hospital care is unresponsive to the access cost and that for GP consultations is the reverse. In other words, people regard stays in hospital as so important that they put aside cost and inconvenience. But in the case of outpatient and GP surgery visits, distance might rule out visits for (apparently) minor complaints – the inconvenience of access may be greater than the inconvenience of the condition. That may not be a cause for concern. On the other hand, it could lead to lower rates of detection of serious illness. As Bentham and Haynes (1984) put it:

> . . . there is a strong possibility that inadequate access to GPs in the remoter rural districts leads to inadequate access to hospital care. (p 85)

Table 7.7 Percentage rates of general practitioner consultations and out patient attendances by area type and population characteristics for persons with long standing illness

Group		GP consultations Urban	Rural	Outpatients Urban	Rural	Subsample size
Age	18-44	52*	31*	62	40	(82)
	45-64	47	34	47	38	(114)
	65+	50*	32*	40	27	(143)
Sex:	Male	45	30	45	33	(147)
	Female	52	35	50	34	(190)
Car:	Car-owning	39	34	46	35	(214)
	Not car-owning	60**	28**	51**	30**	(126)
Social:	Manual	62*	34*	33	37	(138)
	Non-manual	45	31	66**	27**	(136)

* Significant at 0.05;   ** Significant at 0.01

Source: Haynes and Bentham (1982)

The data are not available to decide the issue though there is evidence, cited in Chapter 8, that poor access, in geographical and other terms, does deter hospital use. The evidence presented by Bentham and Haynes does suggest that distance from health facilities is linked to lower levels of use; the issue they are not able to resolve is precisely why the link arises.

Even if distance does not deter, it may still impose clinical costs on patients. The London Renal Services Review argued that 'the need for provision of transport is likely to increase' while the costs – in terms of stress and strain – to the patient of long trips undermined the quality of treatment. As a result, they suggested that tertiary centres are not a good option for most patients: instead satellite services were likely to be more effective. But quantification or even systematic qualitative description of patients' experiences is lacking.

In the case of serious injuries or medical conditions, access may be critical. In the case of cardiac arrest, the critical time is very short and hence a satisfactory response must be provided 'on site', not within the Accident and Emergency Department, either by ambulance staff or members of the public. A number of studies (SHHD 1994) have shown the value, in terms of survival and reduction in neurological complications, of the provision of resuscitation by bystanders – not normally part of the formal care system at all:

... the available evidence suggests that the use of bystander CPR [cardio-pulmonary resuscitation]could double the survival rate of patients who suffer a cardiac arrest outside hospital (though the improvement in survival rates varies considerably from one study to another). (p 25)

The implication of this example is that the critical response times are pre-hospital and may involve non-professionals, rather than time spent getting to hospital. Distance and time taken to hospital are not decisive for those patients who can only benefit from a virtually immediate response. They are helped only by a locally organised response of a kind, such as that provided by the Fire Service in Seattle (Mayer 1979a).

In the case of serious accident and emergencies, it seems reasonable to assume that speed of access to hospital is important in determining the outcome of care. A commonly cited rule of thumb is that, in the case of serious trauma, a gap of over an hour between incident and effective intervention spells danger. The golden hour rule was formulated some 20 years ago and appears to have been based originally on medical intuition rather than careful analysis. For some injuries, it does not hold (Berk *et al*, 1987). Sampalis *et al* (1992), however, found that patients treated within an hour did fare better, but the numbers taking longer than one hour to hospital were small – 13 out of a sample of 270. Furthermore, time was treated dichotomously so the significance of differences in time under one hour was not estimated. However, Pepe *et al* (1987) found no differences in survival rates from penetrating injuries between four time bands – 0-20, 21-30, 31-40 and over 40 minutes. Gervin and Fisher's (1982) study of penetrating heart injuries found time between injury and treatment in hospital of critical importance while on-site treatment reduced chances of survival because of the delay imposed. However, data from the UK Major Trauma Outcome Study (personal communication) appear to suggest that time is not critical to survival. Although the mortality rate rises with severity, it does not rise with time. Indeed, in some cases, the reverse is true: see Table 7.8. This may reflect the fact that the longer access times are associated with some degree of pre-treatment, or that the longer trips involve less seriously ill people. In other words, as with the studies reviewed in Chapter 5, patient selection may have disguised the true effect of time and distance.

Analysis carried out in Seattle (Mayer, 1979b) also found the paradoxical conclusion that shorter response times to incidents did not increase survival chances. Again this might, as the author suggested, be an artefact of the data or of differences imperfectly understood between the type of accidents occurring in different locations. Bentham (1986), using published data

Table 7.8 Time between injury and arrival at hospital with mortality rates

Injury severity score

Interval	1-8	9-15	16-24	25-40	41-49	50-75	Total
<15 mins	429, 2(0.5)	279, 4(1.4)	65, 14(21.5)	67, 38(56.7)	9, 9(100)	12, 10(83.3)	861, 77(11.2)
>15 mins <30 min	1160, 10(0.9)	859, 16(1.9)	195, 31(15.9)	176, 87(49.4)	29, 25(86.2)	34, 32(94.1)	2453, 201(8.2)
>30 mins <60 min	2303, 17(0.7)	1673, 32(1.9)	314, 49(15.7)	267, 102(38.2)	45, 28(62.2)	46, 39(84.8)	4648, 267(5.8)
>1 hr < 2 hr	1274, 14(1.1)	926, 20(2.2)	184, 20(10.9)	177, 73(41.2)	26, 22(84.6)	22, 20(90.0)	2609, 149(5.7)
> 2 hr	955, 18(1.9)	545, 26(4.8)	152, 25(16.4)	138, 52(37.7)	14, 9(64.3)	7, 4(57.1)	1811, 114(6.3)

Note: above = total number of patients, number of deaths(mortality rate)
Source: UK National Trauma Outcome Study

sources relating death from motor vehicle accidents to different types of area, – rural, inner city – and to the availability of an A&E department, found that the risk of death from motor accidents was higher in areas which did not have an emergency facility sited within them and in rural areas whether or not they had one. As Bentham points out, such an analysis is not conclusive but it is at least suggestive that distance increases risk. An alternative possibility is that there is a link between severity and distance which would arise if accidents in rural areas were on average more severe as they would be if they tended to consist of proportionately more road accidents.

Thus the precise relationship between access times and survival chances cannot be pinned down until further detailed studies are carried out. However, it is becoming standard practice in the UK for ambulance crews to be trained in a number of procedures designed to improve the injured person's survival chances. According to a report by the National Audit Office (1992), the current aim is to have one trained paramedic in every emergency ambulance by March 1997 and 'The ultimate aim of the paramedic programme is to provide properly trained staff, vehicles and equipment so that care can begin at the earliest opportunity, with the objective of reducing mortality and morbidity.' A recent study by the National Audit Office in Scotland (1992) also suggested that by extra expenditure, both on the training of paramedics and on better communications between crews and main accident centres, the quality of service could be raised in those remote areas of the country which were a long way from a properly equipped accident and emergency centre. In these ways the inevitable clinical costs of long access times should, the report argues, be reduced. However, this assurance, as well as the Ministerial statement, is not totally supported by the evidence. While again it may seem commonsense that on-site measures are valuable and they undoubtedly are for some patients, such as those who are trapped by debris or who are losing blood rapidly, the evidence is far from clear whether they are for all.

A report on rural emergency services in the US (Office of Technology Assessment, 1989) concluded that some of the measures taken on site were of no proven value:

> *There is no evidence, for example, that the pneumatic antishock garment that is standard on ambulances is effective for victims of penetrating trauma... there is little evidence that endotrachical intubation is useful when performed out of the hospital; and there is some evidence that trying to expedite the administration of medication by starting IV lines in the field is ineffective. (p 47)*

For some patients the delays while paramedics decide what to do or implement some procedures such as IV lines may reduce their chances overall. The traditional scoop and run policies may be best for some classes of patient where the time taken to reach hospital may be critical.

The question then is: where should the ambulance run to? Within a trauma system, patients could go to the nearest accident and emergency facility and then be transferred to the trauma centre itself once a local diagnosis had been carried out to ensure its necessity. That process of transfer itself involves risks, even though in the majority of cases patients can be, and are, transported safely. Ehrenworth *et al* (1986) found that critically ill patients could be safely transported over long distances by special transport teams and long distance transfers are commonplace in sparsely settled areas. But transfer may not be carried out well in practice. An audit of transfer of unconscious head-injured patients to a neuro-surgical unit by Gentleman and Jennett (1990) found that around half were not looked after properly. The safety of transporting patients between – and also within – hospitals cannot be taken for granted in cases of serious head injury, for example, not only because of the transfer itself but also because of the division of responsibility for care.

In general the clinical effects of long-distance transfer or of the costs – including, in the case of inter-hospital transfer, an accompanying doctor – of doing so are poorly evidenced. That in part arises because it is not given systematic attention. The Audit Commission's report (1992) on children's hospital services confirmed that those children requiring transfer were often given little serious attention by either managers or clinicians.

7.3 Conclusion

Overall, it appears that access does pose costs and inconvenience to users of hospital services and may also impose clinical costs, particularly for emergency cases. The former may be severe for some population groups, particularly elderly people, those without a car, and those with dependents. Hence a more concentrated pattern for delivering hospitals would run the risk of reducing overall quality of care. However, that risk seems greatest for outpatient rather than inpatient care. But, leaving home care to one side, no pattern of service delivery will remove all access penalties: so-called local facilities can also be hard to get to.

As far as accident and emergency services are concerned, the relationship between outcome and access time remains to be established for the full range of patients with which they deal. Access times are important for some patients, though not all, nor to the same degree. But most emergency admissions are not accident victims and their lives may not be in immediate danger; they may need close monitoring rather than immediate treatment.

Unless the link can be made between superior performance once patients are treated and the possible losses from enforcing longer trips, then the overall benefits of centralisation of emergency services cannot be identified. Studies cited here do not provide sufficient evidence to demonstrate the form of the relationship between access time and clinical outcome for the range of conditions requiring emergency care. Indeed, some appear to suggest time is not important.

If different thresholds exist for different classes of injury, then benefits to some patients resulting from centralisation may be at the expense of disbenefits to others. Thus for some injuries, access to the full emergency resources of the hospital is important: for others not. The critical issue therefore is how decisions are taken to direct patients to different hospitals and whether decision-making can be improved by, for example, better training or communications links between ambulance and hospital, or better decision-making within the ambulance service itself. Most ambulance services do not attempt to prioritise emergency calls, but recent experiments in the Derbyshire and Essex ambulance services have suggested it can be done. If so, then cases where time may be critical will on average be attended to more quickly.

The overall conclusion which emerges is that the implications of access times for patients as a whole cannot be demonstrated. Some pieces of the required evidence are available: what is missing is a definition of the precise relationship between access times, alternative service patterns and outcomes, for different classes of patient: without that, the merits and demerits of alternative dispositions of hospital emergency services cannot be estimated. The difficulty, however, is not simply lack of evidence; more fundamentally, the evidence reviewed here and elsewhere in more detail (Pencheon, forthcoming) consists of small-scale studies of parts of a number of different emergency services. Any attempt, therefore, to integrate their findings is fraught with difficulty.

That conclusion applies equally to the two preceding chapters. In general, the evidence required to demonstrate the key relationships between quality of care, costs and access is not available. Consequently, the central questions posed at the end of Chapter 1 cannot be answered in a systematic and satisfactory way. The framework for analysis set out in Chapters 3 and 4 cannot, therefore, be converted into a set of simple rules or guidelines. Furthermore,

Chapters 5, 6 and 7 have focused on the areas which appeared most likely to be well evidenced. Some areas, particularly those bearing on the teaching of doctors and the subsequent maintenance and development of their careers have not been addressed. Moreover, the significance of some of the evidence which has been presented is itself undermined by new developments, both in these fields and in medical and information technology which present new opportunities for, as well as threats to, the acute general hospital. To these we turn in the following three chapters.

CHAPTER 8

The demand for hospital services

The context within which hospital planners must work is changing rapidly. A large number of factors are at work which bear on the search for the 'right' balance of activity between hospitals and other providers. Some of these tend to support present patterns of provision by improving the services which the acute hospital has to offer, others to undermine it by making it easier to effect substitution: some forces make for greater concentration, others for dispersal.

This and the following two chapters attempt to show how these factors bear on the central concepts discussed in earlier chapters – clustering, concentration, separability, substitution – and hence how they should influence the future pattern of delivery of hospital services. The present chapter considers the demand or need for hospital services: that both terms are required reflects the fact that the transition to a market framework is not complete. Purchasers will still appropriately think in terms of the needs of their populations for health care, but providers must increasingly think in terms of demand for their services, ie what they can persuade purchasers to pay for and hence how they can, in a world of budget constraints, protect or even enhance their market share. Chapter 9 examines the factors facing the supply of hospital services looking first at medical technology, then at staffing issues, and finally at management structures. Finally, Chapter 10 turns to access, transport and communications, which provide the links between the demand for and supply of hospital services.

8.1 Recent trends and prospects

Until recently, the demand for acute hospital care has appeared open-ended. Activity measured in terms of admissions has risen ever since the formation of the NHS, and its rate of increase shows no sign of diminishing. During the ten years up to 1992/93, activity increased at a little over two per cent per year, but in the 1990s, the increase has been about four per cent, much higher than the growth rate since the 1970s. Although some part of that increase may be ascribed to re-admission of the patients (ie within 30 days of their first admission), most of the increase can be ascribed to a rise in the number of different patients treated: see Table 8.1. Re-admissions have risen, as a proportion of total admissions, but only slightly.

Table 8.1   Trends in re-admissions, Scotland, 1983-1990

	1983	1990
	% Total Admissions	
Emergency re-admission		
After emergency admission	7.5	9.6
After elective admission	2.8	3.7
Elective re-admission		
After emergency admission	2.8	3.1
After elective admission	6.4	7.2

Source: Information and Statistics Division, Scottish Health Service (1993), Trends in hospital re-admission rates in Scotland 1983 to 1990, *Health Briefing No 93/23*

Furthermore, as activity has risen, the numbers waiting for treatment have also risen. At the end of 1994, numbers waiting for treatment exceeded one million, a similar figure to that obtaining at the beginning of the 1980s. Behind the recorded waiting lists, it has been frequently conjectured, lies a 'bottomless pit' of demand for care which would be revealed if waiting lists were to shorten as a result of some sudden upsurge in spending.

The notion of a bottomless pit of demand for care in part derives from waiting list evidence and in part from a belief that if something is free, people will always want more of it. The nature of the metaphor, however, reveals uncertainty as to the factors which in practice shape the demands for hospital services. Economic, demographic and technological factors, as well as the health status of the population, clearly play a role but it is hard to isolate their individual effects. It is clear, however, that most of the increase in activity during the 1980s cannot be accounted for by changes in demography.

For much of the 1980s, debate about the adequacy of the NHS budget was conducted with reference to demographic and technological change. As far as the first of these is concerned, the Department of Health regularly published an estimate of the extra resources needed to cope with changes in the age composition of the population. This usually was less than one per cent per year, lower than the actual rate of increase in activity.

The Department does not concede that there is any necessary link between their estimate of the impact of demographic change and the NHS budget; the emphasis is now on raising productivity. Nevertheless, it continues to press for higher levels of activity, as measured by finished consultant episodes. This pressure does not, however, result from any attempt to understand and forecast what the future role of the hospital should be. The NHS has never attempted to meet a forecast demand: instead, it has aimed to make best use of whatever resources the Government has made available to it, in the light of the number and type of patients who present themselves for treatment. And that level of resources is not itself the result of a systematic analysis of the market the NHS hospital serves.

Most projections of the demand for hospital services made for the purposes of planning new capacity have tended to assume that growth would continue more of less as in the past and that in turn has been influenced primarily by the availability of finance to the NHS. Availability of finance turns on growth in the national economy. Assuming a continued growth in GDP, further growth in spending within the NHS might be expected; there is a strong relationship between income and spending on health care across a wide range of countries. On this basis, continued GDP growth would seem to guarantee further growth in demand for hospital services.

8.2 Some aspects of overall demand

The notion of the overall demand for hospital services, however, is essentially a shorthand way of referring to the demand for a wide range of different activities. Indeed, the very heterogeneity of hospital work means that it is impractical to consider each and every element in a survey of this kind. Instead, the rest of this chapter considers a small number of areas which impinge critically on the way that hospitals are organised and their role in the health care sector as a whole:

- changes in the composition of need
- routes to hospital
- consumer preferences
- the scope for substitution
- markets which should be conceded.

Changes in the composition of need

The main threat to the hospital, it is sometimes argued, arises from a change in the nature of demand for health care, away from what hospitals are best at, towards services where other care providers have a comparative advantage. Infectious diseases, once a main user of hospital beds, are now of minor importance, while the very success of certain hospital procedures in prolonging life, as well as of some preventive measures taken outside the hospital, have led to a growing need for continuing care, which is primarily a matter for services outside hospitals rather than the episodic care in which they are increasingly specialising.

The significance of this change is that the links with the community grow in importance relative to those within the hospital. That has, as argued in Chapter 4, important implications for the organisation of care, but it also has implications for its content, tilting the balance of advantage away from the type of services where hospitals are most appropriate to those where other forms of care delivery are competitive.

As far as infectious diseases are concerned, it may be, as a number of doctors have warned (Garrett, 1994) that the unexpected will happen. The emergence of AIDS and the re-emergence of diseases such as tuberculosis which appeared to have been virtually eliminated, points up the inherent uncertainty that must attach to any forecast of what the health care system of the next century will have to deal with. In early 1994, *The Economist* (1994a) set out a scenario plotting the spread of a fictitious disease from an Asian source to a world-wide pandemic claiming half a million lives a year in its first summer. 'The journey from obscurity to pandemic was tortuous, but each step was stunningly ordinary.' The scenario serves to underline the weakness of any demand forecast, but as of now, there appears no specific possibility against which to plan. The lesson of the article and Garrett's monumental study is that that could quickly change.

Infectious diseases no longer absorb a significant share of hospital resources. Treatment of chronic or progressive conditions do. Patients with chronic conditions may require hospital treatment, eg in the case of asthma collapse, even though the bulk of their needs is already met by GPs, community nurses and social care providers. With better care outside hospital, including better self-care, hospital use may be diminished. But the opposite may also be true. Elective interventions can reduce demands on other providers of care, including both health and social services, as well as restoring mobility to the patient. Thus cataract surgery appears to be both effective from the viewpoint of the patient and economically beneficial in terms of saving public sector long term care costs (Williams *et al*, 1992). In neither case does the long term, progressive nature of the condition preclude an effective role for the hospital.

The same is true of the ageing population. The elderly currently make up about half the work-load of the hospital measured in terms of bed days. They use hospital services more intensively than other age groups and their treatment rates have been rising faster than average: see Table 8.2. Their numbers, or more precisely the numbers of very elderly people who are the heaviest users of hospitals, are set to increase; demand would seem set to rise.

Table 8.2   Hospitalisation rates per 1,000 population: Scotland

| | Males | | | | |
	0-44	45-64	65-74	75-84	85+
1981	88.0	143.9	241.8	299.5	319.9
1992	116.6	222.1	401.2	492.7	544.9
% Increase	132.5	154.3	165.9	164.5	170.3
	Females				
	0-44	45-64	65-74	75-84	85+
1981	97.0	127.2	167.6	209.9	234.1
1992	132.0	201.3	277.0	331.3	368.0
% Increase	136.1	158.3	165.3	157.8	157.2

Source: Management Executive, NHS in Scotland, (1994a)

But should we expect treatment rates to rise? It has been argued, most forcefully by Fries (1989), that longer life should be accompanied by a longer period of freedom from ill health. The most extreme version of this view is reflected in the so-called triangulation or compression hypothesis – see Diagram 8.1 – which, if correct, would imply a falling demand for health care among the very elderly. In the form Fries puts it, the compression hypothesis combines an assumption of an upper limit to average length of life – shown as 80 in the diagram – and a shortening of the period before death of chronic or severe morbidity. The alternative, shown as scenario I, combines an upper limit with a lengthening period of morbidity. Scenario II shows the reverse.

However, the evidence, though far from perfect, does not on balance support Fries as to where the upper limit lies, even though, according to Nesse and Williams (1995), it is reasonable to assume one. Life expectancy appears to be continuing to rise, and the period of ill health lengthening rather than shortening. Table 8.3, derived from the *General Household Survey*, shows recent changes in the ratio of expectation of life without disability and life expectancy. If Fries were right, then the value of this ratio would be approaching 100. Instead, it was more or less constant between 1976 and 1985 for women under 75 and hence, as life expectancy was rising, so the period of life with disability has been growing. For both men and women over 75, however, the ratio rose during that period.

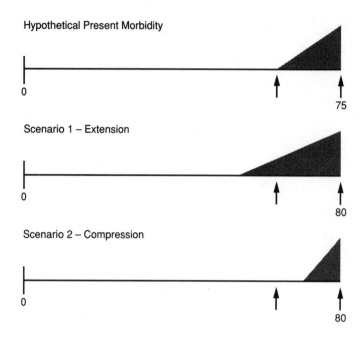

Diagram 8.1. Compression or extension of morbidity?

Table 8.3 Ratio of expectation of life without disability and life expectancy: England and Wales 1976-1985

Age	1976	1981	1985
Men
0	83	82	82
5	82	81	81
15	80	79	79
45	68	68	67
65	55	59	58
75	46	51	52
Women
0	81	79	79
5	80	77	78
15	77	75	75
45	65	62	64
65	50	47	51
75	39	36	41

Source: Bebbington (1988)

Disability is not a direct measure of use of health services: there are no regular data series which monitor how the use of health services of particular individuals changes as they age. Some recent evidence from small-scale studies suggests that those who live longer are the 'healthy survivors'. Bowling *et al* (1994) examined the change in service use among a sample of people aged 85 and over, the first such survey of its kind in the UK. Those who had died between the two years of the survey had been those with poorer functional ability, and use of health and social services was positively correlated with functional ability. Nevertheless, use did increase among those who survived in the period between the two surveys so even the 'healthy survivors' required more care.

As far as hospital services in particular are concerned, Cartwright (1991) found substantial changes in the use of hospitals or other institutions in the year before death, a period when hospital use is at its most intense. As Table 8.4 shows, the proportion spending the whole year before death institutionalised rose from 9 to 15 per cent between 1969 and 1987 while those spending no time in hospital almost halved.

Table 8.4 Length of time in hospital or other institutions in the year before death

	1969 (%)	1987 (%)
Not at all	30	16
Less than one week	12	15
One week but less than a month	21	23
One month but less than three months	19	21
Three months but less than six months	7	6
Six months but less than a year	2	4
A year or more	9	15
Number of deaths (= 100%)	781	631

Source: Cartwright (1991)

The shifts described in Table 8.4 probably reflect changes in medical technology which have made it possible for older people with multiple pathologies to be treated safely in ways which were not feasible even a few years ago. Anticipating the next chapter, it seems likely that further increases will be possible since surgical and anaesthetic techniques will almost certainly be less invasive in future than they are now. But it may also reflect better identification of needs either by better organised general practice or by patients themselves becoming more aware of the potential for treatment. Bowling's work already cited found a significant number of people with poor functional ability – generally a good predictor of service use – who made little use of health services. These may form a latent need group which changes in technology and improvements to primary care will help become 'effective demanders'.

However, treatment rates also depend on the broader social context. It is frequently alleged, for example, that far less is done for elderly people than could be done on current technology because the implicit rationing inherent in the NHS is biased against them. To the extent that this is true and there is evidence for it (Grimley Evans, 1993), eg in respect of the installation of more advanced pacemakers, and becomes recognised by purchasers, then treatment rates for the elderly might grow even further.

On the other hand, as Manton (1991) points out, those currently growing old have enjoyed advantages over their predecessors:

> *It is evident that there are factors that could improve the aggregate health and functioning of the oldest-old population – thereby reducing LTC service needs on a per capita basis. Some factors are associated with past life experiences of the birth cohorts constituting future oldest-old populations. The educational level of those cohorts will increase...Their income and assets will improve on average (there are subgroups disadvantaged on multiple economic and health factors....Future oldest-old cohorts will have had regular medical care for most of their life, lived in environments with reduced public health hazards (e.g., childhood immunization programs; nutritional supplementation; programs against smoking and drinking), and will have had a heightened health awareness possibly leading to improved levels of physical activity and dietary control...the future occupational and social environment of the elderly may be more "tolerant" to physical impairment, allowing future oldest-old populations to better preserve their social and economic autonomy. (p 324)*

All this, of course, is highly speculative: that it should be so reflects the massive difficulties involved in trying to understand the links between ageing and morbidity on the one hand and, on the other, in determining how factors outside the field of health care, such as housing and social support, shape demand for hospital services, as well as policies such as health promotion which also might help to extend the length of 'disability-free' life.

Routes to hospital

As things currently stand, for all but accident and emergency departments and a few other specialised services, individuals cannot gain direct access to hospital services. GPs act as gatekeepers, either to specialists within hospitals or, in a few parts of the country, to beds under their own control. Thus, as far as outpatient services are concerned and any subsequent treatment that is given, hospitals are in the hands of other providers. As far as numbers of outpatient visits are concerned, growth has been much lower than for inpatient activity: from 35.5 million attendances in 1981 to 39.3 in 1994/95.

Despite a great deal of research effort, how the referral process works is to some degree a mystery. As a recent review by Coulter (1992) puts it:

Most studies of referral rates reveal wide variations between practices or between individual practitioners which cannot be explained by differences in morbidity patterns. (p 98)

However, Coulter also suggests (Roland and Coulter, 1992) that despite the observed variation in referral rates, there is no general reason to believe that people are being under- or over-referred to hospital. However, there is evidence for particular conditions. In the case of hernia repair, for example, the Health Care Evaluation Unit at the University of Bristol (1992) found unmet needs because GPs sometimes fail to refer patients for a consultant opinion. As far as the future is concerned, the belief has developed that as general practice is strengthened, it will come to make less use of the hospital. But, as noted in Chapter 4, qualitative arguments point both ways: more effective general practice and better informed patients could reduce hospital referrals, eg for asthma, but could equally well increase them, eg for those conditions such as need for hernia repair, which appears to be underdiagnosed.

The studies surveyed by Roland and Coulter concentrated on referral to outpatient clinics for diagnosis and consultation. However, most medical inpatient admissions bypass this route. Patients are referred directly into hospital by their general practitioner or they refer themselves via the accident and emergency department. Despite their importance to the workload of the hospital, there has been until recently very little analysis of the circumstances under which such referrals are made. This represents a massive gap in understanding the workload of the hospital.

Over the past year or so, a number of hospitals have reported substantial increases in emergency medical admissions. The rise has occurred across all age groups, so neither demographic factors nor the introduction of the community care elements of the NHS and Community Care

Table 8.5 Daily variations in hospital admissions, England 1991/92

Av = 100

	Emergency	Elective
Monday	115	154
Tuesday	109	140
Wednesday	110	141
Thursday	105	126
Friday	127	88
Saturday	80	11
Sunday	76	38

Source: King's Fund Policy Institute

Table 8.6 Monthly variations in hospital admissions, England 1991/92

Av = 100

	Emergency	Elective
January	104	101
February	97	101
March	127	121
April	95	95
May	95	89
June	97	106
July	99	105
August	94	90
September	96	101
October	99	103
November	99	106
December	101	83

Source: As above

Act 1990 appear to be significant influences. Other possible explanations, such as GP fund-holders attempting to get 'free' access for their patients, do not seem to hold. Analysis of emergency admissions at six hospital trusts (Harrison *et al*, 1995) found that all had experienced a surge in admissions during 1993 and early 1994 with respiratory problems, and a steady rise in cardiac diagnoses. The first might be related to environmental conditions, though no such link has in fact been demonstrated; the second could be attributed to a greater awareness on the part of GPs of the value of early treatment with streptokinase. Other studies have suggested other explanations (Edwards and Warneke 1994; Kendrick 1995). Already, in conjunction with the rapid growth in day care, growth in emergency care is altering significantly the balance of hospital inpatient activity. As a consequence, the importance of unplanned use is growing relative to planned, and hence the workload of the hospital is becoming inherently more variable and harder to predict.

In Chapter 2, it was argued that it is generally more economic to pool variable demands, and so any shift of this sort would tend to improve the economics of larger units, or create a case for managing demand over larger areas where geography allows this, ie effectively running beds in different locations as one pool, in the way in which the Emergency Bed Service in London and similar institutions in other cities work. There is, however, very little published information about the variability of demand for emergency care on an inpatient basis nor indeed about its nature and the factors underlying it. Hospital episode statistics can provide some insight into its nature.

Emergency inflows are generally lower at weekends – see Table 8.5 – and there are also variations between different times of year – see Table 8.6. With one or two exceptions, such as the March peak, the variations shown here are not massive and some, such as the higher than average elective inflows on Mondays and Wednesdays, readily predictable. But at the level of the individual hospital much wider variations may occur. Harrison *et al* plotted the number of occasions emergency admissions in one of the hospitals they studied were more than one standard deviation away from the moving average calculated over four weeks. In one year, 15 exceptional in flows were recorded and 12 in the next.

A better understanding of the pattern of utilisation and the factors underlying it is required if the case for strengthening the capacity of hospitals to handle emergency admission is to be properly made. It is not just a question of bed numbers, but also of the availability of experienced staff, particularly for urgent consultation or diagnosis (Coast *et al*, 1995) as well as facilities outside the hospital itself. Also, since the lower the degree of acceptable risk of hospitals not being able to meet peak demands, the higher the cost of provision, the stronger the case for examining the scope for preventing some admissions by suitable responses by other providers. At present, an emergency response outside the acute hospital, other than through GPs, is only available in one or two part of the country, run by community trusts on an experimental, or small-scale, basis. These suggest that for some classes of patient, ie those whose needs are for temporary support, which family and GP are in combination unable to supply, a service provided by community nurses is effective as least in certain circumstances but more work needs to be done to demonstrate their role within the overall response of the NHS to emergencies.

Consumer preferences

For most of the post-war period, users of the NHS have been patients rather than consumers, fortunate recipients of whatever providers provided. That has begun to change. During the 1980s, there has been a general shift towards a more consumer-oriented service. That has led to, or been reflected in the *Patient's Charter*, and, at local level, attempts to involve users in discussions about the way that care should be provided.

The issue, however, goes deeper than preference for a particular way of delivering hospital care. It also concerns different styles of care, particularly the role of the patient in deciding what care should be delivered and what the patient's role in the process of decision should be. So it is not just a matter of how patients react to different treatment options but also how they might respond if they knew in advance what the implications of different courses of action or inaction might be. It is also a matter of what is sometimes called the care model: the hospital as it stands now is generally based on the so-called medical model, within which the task is to find a specific treatment for a specific condition. Alternative models stress social and psychological aspects as determinants of the need for and the form of care as well as elements that may be valued in the process of care itself.

Whatever the model, the behaviour of the individual may still have some independent impact, be that at the stage of deciding whether to consult a GP or subsequently to press for, or accept, a hospital appointment. How these decisions are made is imperfectly understood, but there is evidence that the way the options available are presented to patients will influence the course of treatment chosen.

As Kasper *et al* (1992) point out:

> *Most medical conditions have multiple treatments, some with very different benefits and harms.*

So far only a modest amount of work to inform patients of the implications of alternative forms of treatment has been done in this country, but in the US, there are indications that the impact is considerable. It appears (Kasper *et al*, 1992) that reductions of between 44 and 60 per cent in prostatectomy rates have been observed: those responsible for developing the

Table 8.8   Patients' opinions on travelling for treatment

Months	1	2	3	6	12	24
% preferring to travel than wait (months)	34.4	53.8	72.2	88.7	96.1	97.2

Source: Stewart and Donaldson (1991)

programme have found that in respect of benign prostatic hyperplasia it tends to shift preferences towards 'watchful waiting' and away from the active intervention of the surgical option.

Thus the choices made by an informed patient may be different from one who follows professional advice. But at the moment, the evidence on the possible scale of that effect is limited not least because of the narrow range of conditions for which programmes have been

Table 8.9   Waiting list times that patients would tolerate before preferring to travel for operation (113 patients)

Waiting list time (months)	1	2	3	6	9	12	18	24
No. preferring to travel	44	49	60	84	92	103	104	113

Source: Howell et al (1990)

Table 8.10   Distances that patients would be willing to travel for operation (113 patients)

Miles(km)	50(80)	100(160)	200(320)	300(480)
No. willing to travel	102	88	75	75

Source: Howell et al (1990)

developed. That reflects not only the novelty of the technique but also the limited range of conditions for which satisfactory information on the merits of alternative courses of treatment is available to deploy it.

Within the framework set out in Chapter 2, a critical area of choice is between access costs and quality of care. Because quality differences between hospitals are not generally recognised in the UK, choices of this kind have not been studied extensively. However, there is

Table 8.11   Patients' attitude to travel for earlier appointment

	No. of respondents	No further	Up to 10 miles	Up to 30 miles	More than 30 miles
Specialist orthopaedic					
1991	152	42.1	18.4	13.8	25.7
1992	130	40.8	20.8	17.7	20.8
Specialist ophthalmology					
1991	461	47.7	26.9	7.4	18.0
1992	170	54.7	22.3	10.0	12.9
District general hospital: 1					
1991	207	34.3	46.8	10.6	8.2
1992	419	32.9	42.5	16.2	8.3
Teaching hospital					
1991	473	36.2	41.0	10.1	12.7
1992	336	32.4	49.4	8.9	9.3
District general hospital: 2					
1991	216	33.3	44.5	10.6	11.6
1992	331	29.9	49.5	8.5	12.1

Source: Mahon et al (1994)

evidence that people are willing to travel long distances to get treatment earlier than they might otherwise have obtained it. A study of patients offered treatment outside their district of residence (Stewart and Donaldson, 1991) to reduce waiting list times found that most were happy with the experience:

> The results of this study have shown that patients with relatively straightforward surgical problems without any coexisting morbidity are keen to travel to have the problem dealt with quickly. (p 509)

The patients studied by Stewart and Donaldson were offered transport by taxi or minibus and the journeys ranged from 35 to 55 miles. Eighty four per cent of patients needing surgery opted to travel. They report an 'after' survey of those participating in the scheme which shows it to have been highly successful: 98.9 per cent thought travelling schemes to be a good idea. They also reveal an *ex post* relationship between time waiting and willingness to participate: by six months, the vast majority said they would have preferred to travel: see table. 8.8.

These results agree closely with a similar study (Howell *et al*, 1990) where the journeys were 120 miles. In this study, only half accepted the offer of earlier treatment at the cost of extra travel, though they were offered minibus or car transport to make their journey easier. But of those that did only four said they would not want to travel again – though a much larger number found the return trip uncomfortable. Table 8.9 mirrors the previous one, showing people's willingness to travel against wait and distance: the numbers fall, but not dramatically. Table 8.10 shows the reported impact of distance.

Other studies have found people to be more reluctant to travel. Mahon *et al* (1994) found, among a sample of predominantly older people that just over one third were unwilling to travel far for treatment: see Table 8.11.

They found, however, that willingness to travel varied as between specialties – though not diagnostic group – and also with age. Recognising the conflict with other evidence, they point out that their respondents were '. . . suffering from conditions which may well have affected their ability to travel'. They conclude by saying that:

> *These findings suggest that patients cannot been seen as a homogeneous group and that willingness to travel depends on the type of services that patients are seeking, so that those seeking more specialist care which may not be available locally reported a greater willingness to travel, while patients referred for treatment that is or should be available locally are less willing to travel. (p 122)*

If this is right, then willingness to travel turns on expectations of the kind of service that ought to be in place and hence will be modified in response to what actually is available.

Another source of evidence about the impact of travel is that collected by Cullis *et al* (1981) in the late 1970s on visits to outpatients in different locations. Here the choice lay between a longer trip and an earlier appointment on the one hand and a shorter trip and a delayed appointment on the other. Again, the findings were mixed with some preferring to trade distance with speed of access and others the reverse.

These findings suggest that willingness to travel turns on a number of circumstances – length of wait, expectations about local facilities, physical condition and mode of travel. Because people value or disvalue these factors in differing degrees, different choices emerge. If this is so, then to some degree choice could be affected by altering the conditions under which choice was made, eg by altering the transport element in the choices offered, or more fundamentally the information available to users.

Overall, the evidence suggests that people's willingness to trade access off against other aspects of care varies. There is, of course, every reason to expect that people will have different views because of their state of health, family circumstances and the transport options open to them. But if so, then the clear implication is that there will not be agreement on the acceptability of changes affecting the location of hospitals.

However, results of the kind reported here reflect people's current experience or perception of access and the benefits of making longer trips. If the attitudes are to some extent conventional, reflecting expectations of where services should be, they may be susceptible to change in response to new forms of service delivery. The favourable results obtained by Stewart and Donaldson may in part be due to the fact that dedicated transport services were laid on for the patients concerned, and in this way the effective choices facing patients were changed. Within the hospital sector as it stands, differences in the quality of care, broadly defined, may arise.

Choices may involve perceptions of different degrees of risk: some patients may be prepared to trade the risk of poor quality outcomes against other aspects of care. A study (Phibbs *et al* 1993) of the choices made by women of place of delivery found that high-risk women were more influenced by outcome factors while:

> *Although low risk women do not ignore quality, they tend to place less emphasis on the outcome-oriented quality factors. ... which is consistent with their low-risk status. These mothers seem to place more emphasis on factors perceived to influence the "ambience" of the birth experience. (p 218).*

Although these findings come from maternity care, the issue of risk runs right through consideration of the merits of different configurations of hospital services. At present, judgements as to what is 'safe' are largely in the hands of professionals – individual clinicians and the Royal Colleges. As relative risks are poorly documented, there is no way of knowing how people respond to them in practice, and hence how willing or unwilling they would be to trade risk of a poor clinical outcome against access.

In the UK a number of studies, reviewed by Higgins (1993), have suggested that people prefer small to large hospitals, in terms of overall satisfaction and with particular reference to the level of communication between patients and staff. Given the Audit Commission's findings (1994) on communications within hospitals, that is scarcely surprising, as the following extract from the report indicates:

91. *The gaps, overlaps, inconsistencies and contradictions in clinical communication only become clear when the hospital is examined from the patient's point of view. Some problems can be resolved comparatively easily because the changes required – such as re-wording standard letters of appointment to give disabled patients information about access, or making sure information about the national voluntary organisations that specialise in helping patients with particular conditions is posted – are comparatively simple.*

92. *Other problems are more difficult to resolve because they are linked to the culture of the hospital, to the organisation of care and to traditional relationships between professions. If prostate patients, for instance, are going to hear about retrograde ejaculation and other complications before agreeing to surgery, some consultants and clinical teams need to change their approach to communication. Some gaps in information for patients will only be filled when groups of staff that currently do not communicate with each other, begin to do so.*

However, these findings are only a starting point, since it may be possible for hospitals to make themselves more attractive to patients and thus to some degree can affect the 'competitive' balance by modifying the way that hospital services themselves are delivered within the hospital so as to adapt them to users' requirements, ranging from better organisation of outpatient services to new forms of services.

The underlying point is that the characteristics of each mode of care are in part inherent and in part responsive to management action. Hospitals cannot reproduce home surroundings but many of the criticisms made by users, ranging from the quality of food to the quality of information can be met by appropriate action.

As indicated by the Expert Committee on Maternity Care (Department of Health, 1994) set up in response to the House of Commons Health Committee report on maternity care, women are interested in choice, continuity and control. British hospitals have consistently denied them all three. The hospital cannot reproduce the circumstances of a home delivery, and in that area is not competitive. Nevertheless it can alter the way care is provided so as to increase its chances of satisfying those values by offering choices within the hospital mode, eg midwife-run wards within the hospital itself and offering continuity of personnel and control through the provision of information.

Another example is that of terminal care. Here survey evidence (Dunlop and Davies, 1989) has shown that terminal patients and their families display a range of preferences which may change over the period of the terminal illness. However, 'mode split' will in part depend on the way in which hospitals and other providers organise care for dying patients. The hospice movement developed in part because hospitals were poor providers in this area, but in recent years, a large number of terminal care support teams have been set up (Dunlop and Hockley, 1989) within hospital specifically to address the needs of the dying and their families. Bircumshaw (1993) suggests that formation of such teams does not itself guarantee an appropriate pattern of care but clearly there is scope for hospitals to adapt how they look after the terminally ill.

A more general approach to adapting the hospital to the needs and wishes of the user is the patient-focused hospital. Although this has been promoted as a means of saving costs, its underlying rationale is to make hospitals more 'user-friendly' by reducing the number of parts of the hospital with which patients need to have contact. This in turn requires 'multi-skilling' and physical re-arrangement of the location of equipment, eg by bringing more diagnostic equipment and therapy services to the ward.

According to a report by RKW Partners (1993), patient-focused hospitals offer a number of benefits to patients:

- more personalised care
- less disruption and delay
- clear responsibilities
- more predictable care
- more sensitive organisation of the patient's day.

However, the report also points out that patient-focused care is 'no quick fix. Sustained commitment and leadership is needed over a long period.' And it will involve expenditure upfront without clear and confident expectation of savings to come.

Mode substitution

The potential for locational and mode substitution noted in Chapter 4 derives in part from the preferences people may have for good access, in part from mode-specific qualities and in part from the growing realisation that some activities are clinically separable from the hospital itself.

Alternative ways of providing what have traditionally been hospital services have been introduced in several parts of the country (Hughes and Gordon, 1992). These transfers have been achieved to different locations and for different groups of patients: they have involved, for example, specialist orthopaedic home care teams, who make it possible for patients to return quicker to their homes, and the creation of new options such as home births which are subsequently chosen by some women in preference to hospital delivery.

Transfers such as these represent what was termed above a series of salami slices off the current hospital workload, as individuals or groups in particular areas have seen and taken specific opportunities to change both the locus of care and also the locus of responsibility. In many cases, 'hospital at home' schemes essentially represent accelerated discharge. By allowing patients to be discharged more quickly than they otherwise would, they 'cut off' some of the inpatient stay, but not the treatment phase. In other cases, such as nutritional therapies, treatment itself is transferred to the home setting, but such examples are few.

These examples largely involve those activities identified in Chapter 3 as potentially separable or substitutable because the clinical links to other hospital activities are weak. They have emerged from local rather than national initiatives. They have not emerged from a detailed examination of each element of the workload of the hospital nor of the implications for the hospital of such transfers.

The closest approach to such an examination, at least in the UK, has been carried out in Bromley. This study (Spiby *et al*, 1995) identified the scope for transfer of activity away from the district general hospital taking diagnosis by diagnosis in a number of clinical areas. The authors of this study stress, however, that the results do not necessarily apply to other areas since they reflect local facilities and local views.

An alternative approach to that adopted in Bromley used by the present authors, has been to take a particular user group and consider how they might be provided with care in a less hospital-dependent way. Drawing on evidence presented to the House of Commons Health Select

Committee and from Audit Commission reports, Harrison and Prentice (1994) were able to show that sufficient evidence and experience existed to support a switch, for some patients, in the mode of care. In the case of children, for example, where the case for minimising hospital stays has been accepted for 30 years at least, a number of instances were identified where hospital care had been transferred to other settings, some involving GPs, and others, community paediatric nurses, but these examples were not typical of the country as a whole.

What neither this, nor any other study has done, is to answer how far that shift might be taken. Murphy (1994) has presented an analysis of an alternative pattern of care for the elderly which took as its starting premiss the aim of reducing the use of hospital facilities. The analysis is essentially structured in three parts: preventing admissions, reducing time spent in hospital if admitted, and developing alternative forms of care delivery.

Preventing admissions

According to her analysis:

> At present, in far too many districts patients are 'sent up to accident and emergency' for assessment, which may result in inappropriate admissions. The hospital based junior doctors usually responsible for the initial assessment of such patients rarely have sufficient experience to have a good overview of what community-based treatments might be offered and the 'hole in the community' closes up very swiftly when a sick older person vacates the fragile tenure of their home support system. (p 67)

On the basis of such an assessment – or possibly just on the basis of the GP's own – an emergency response can be provided in the home setting. At present,

> these schemes tend to be one-off innovations by local enthusiasts which are not sufficiently comprehensive to make a district-wide impact on the use of beds. (p 71)

Alternatively, hospitals themselves can provide assessment facilities so as to analyse what is needed before formal admission. A number of hospitals are now using pre-admission wards which delay the decision to admit until it is clear that inpatient care actually is required.

Focusing on the elderly, Murphy suggests, in the article referred to above, a number of measures which might be used to reduce the incidence of emergency admissions:

Box 8.1: Measures to reduce the incidence of emergency admissions

■ Review all patients taking night sedation

■ See all patients taking more than three drugs to review the necessity for them

■ Identify all elderly people who smoke and give direct advice

■ Identify all women under 45-52kg, men under 55kg, women over 70kg and men over 75-80kg in order to assess the malnourished and give advice on obesity

■ Incorporate a question on mood state into 75+ check to detect depression and devise a specific care plan to tackle it

■ Visit all patients recently discharged from hospital to assess their care plan

■ Screen elderly people for hypertension and treat it

■ Check all 75+ for vision, hearing and foot care and ensure appropriate aids and services are provided

■ Prescribe aspirin to those suspected of having myocardial infarction or stroke

■ Identify those whose cognitive impairment has become evident to relatives and neighbours and carry out a full assessment of the patient's and their carers' needs

see Box 8.1. How effective these are remains to be demonstrated by experience on the ground.

Why the emergencies arise in the first place and hence whether they can be prevented is not understood. There is very little information to go on: as noted already, although most medical cases treated in hospital represent emergency admissions, very little is known as to why they occur. In the case of asthma, it seems many are due to patients and their doctors not being familiar with the signs which would indicate an oncoming attack of a severity requiring admission. A study by Blainey et al (1990) of hospital admissions of asthma patients, the numbers of which have been rising, found that many patients did not receive the treatment immediately prior to admission that would have avoided the need to enter hospital. In some cases, entry was unavoidable, as the attacks were too sudden. In others, the signs had been present for some time and in some cases GPs' advice had been sought. The authors conclude that both patients and their doctors need educating in the scope for preventive measures which could reduce hospital use.

Reducing time in hospital

Some measures apply right across the board to all care groups, ie better bed management and discharge procedures. To get the full value out of these, Murphy argues, requires guidelines covering the whole process of care and involving all the relevant professionals. At present no such guidelines exist across the full clinical range. In the case of community hospitals, that may mean that lengths of stay are much higher than they need be for lack of a proper management regime. In the case of acute hospitals, it may mean that beds are persistently blocked because patients cannot be moved out to small local units or because a system of home support cannot be put in place quickly enough, or with the appropriate type of professional support.

Providing alternatives

As Murphy notes, hospitals are used 'because they are there' and because there has been no attempt systematically to find alternatives to them. In some areas such as Inner London, long term care facilities are in short supply because of the cost of suitably priced properties. They may have to be created. In others, the obstacles are of different kinds. The accident and emergency department, like the police station, is a 24-hour facility and both attract custom they would prefer not to have, because other facilities such as social services observe formal weekday hours even if their clients do not and GP surgeries are also typically closed most evenings and weekends. But this need not to be so: issues of 'turf' to one side, it is easy enough to imagine an emergency facility based in a health centre, serving a small part of the catchment area of a large hospital. That could have all the facilities required to avert the admission of some elderly patients.

Several points emerge from this analysis: first, none of the proposals turn on technological developments which are not yet proven. In that sense, the various ideas and possibilities Murphy discusses are currently feasible – though that is not to say they are worthwhile, taking all things into account.

Second, the obstacles to change lie in professional, financial and organisational boundaries which have up to now prevented a coherent and comprehensive analysis of how to supply services across all providers or, when such an analysis is carried out, rule out some options as non-feasible. For example, any major shift of work to general practice runs up against the unwillingness of GPs to accept it under the existing financial regulation for general medical services, a point returned to below. Furthermore, the majority of district level purchasers continue to contract with specific providers, rather than for broadly defined services to which several providers might contribute.

Third, as demonstrated in Chapters 3 to 7, most of the hard data required to test the cost and clinical implications of different configurations are lacking. This makes change hard to justify except on an experimental and piece-meal basis. Moreover, the absence of data for the same individuals over different parts of the same care episode within the same organisation, and of course over the episodes provided by others, means that a clear picture of what is happening now is not available. In the case of the elderly or the chronically ill, the number of different patterns of 'care career' is not known, ie the numbers of occasional and very frequent users and, among the latter, the mix of services they call on. The broad features of the 'market' to be served cannot be established from routinely available data.

Over ten years ago, Evans (1984) concluded that:

> *No-one has yet attempted to assemble the literature on alternatives to conventional inpatient care, to see what the aggregate impact could be. A study which looked, diagnosis by diagnosis, at the savings in hospital use which have been demonstrated in some form of experimental or*

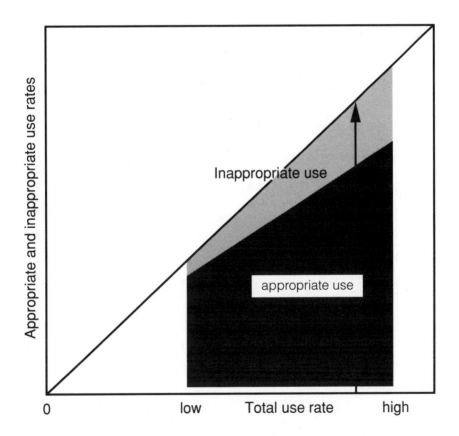

Diagram 8.2 The RAND result (Park 1993)

field trial, without deterioration of patient outcome, would most certainly yield very large numbers indeed (p 197).

That remains true. Although as even the brief selection from the literature drawn on in the chapter indicates, the potential for mode substitution is widely recognised, a systematic working through of the options remains to be carried out in terms which possible competitors of the hospital can readily apply across the full range of possibilities.

Markets which should be conceded

It was argued in Chapter 4 that the roles of hospitals to other providers of care were not clearly distinct. Within these areas which, currently at least, are seen as the preserve of the hospital, the implicit assumption so far has been that what is done in the hospital is of value. But because of the lack of outcome measures for the vast majority of the work done in hospitals, rigorous evidence is not available to confirm or refute that assumption. The proportion of hospital work validated by randomised control trials is low – perhaps 20 per cent. Much will never be because it is too late to carry them out. A large number of studies in different countries have established that rates of intervention vary between different areas for reasons which do not relate to the condition of the patient. But it is hard to determine from work of this kind whether, in the words of Wennberg's famous article (1987), services are rationed in New Haven or over-utilised in Boston. But, in some cases, evidence of ineffectiveness exists, yet procedures concerned continue to be carried out. One such example is dilatation and curettage (Coulter *et al*, 1993).

It is also possible that worthwhile interventions are being performed in inappropriate circumstances. What counts as inappropriate care is not easy to establish and there are no universally agreed conventions. However, according to a series of RAND studies carried out in the US a large proportion of certain operations – 65 per cent of carotid endarterectomies, 28 per cent of upper gatrointestinal endoscopies and 28 per cent of coronary angiographies were done for less than appropriate reasons (Brook, 1993).

Given the high rates of intervention in the US relative to the UK, this may not seem too surprising to a British audience. But application of the same approach to the Trent region of England produced similar results: 51 per cent of coronary angiographies and 42 per cent of CABGs were judged to have been performed for less than appropriate reasons. Thus the RAND approach suggests (Peake, 1993) that inappropriate use is common in all areas, whether these be areas of high or low intervention rates but, as would be expected, that the scale of inappropriate use is greater in the higher use areas: see Diagram 8.2.

Such studies are rare: in England, the Confidential Enquiry into Peri-Operative Deaths has recently highlighted some operations judged inappropriate by its compilers. The 1991/92 report, for example, found some operations done without any realistic hope of success, eg amputations done on patients destined to die within a few days. By its nature the Enquiry does not lend itself to general conclusions about the overall scale of inappropriateness so it is, therefore, not possible to determine, on the basis of the evidence it provides, what share of hospital activity should be put into that category.

8.3 Conclusion

The market for hospital services within the UK health care system is poorly understood, not least because, until now, there has been little incentive to understand it as a market. Hospitals have been content to passively receive the custom referred to them by general practitioners and patients themselves. That will have to change. In the case of emergency admissions, pressures to improve performance on a day-to-day basis require a better understanding of the scale and nature of variations in daily and monthly inflows, as well as the determinants of long term trends. Some of the markets currently served by hospital providers are vulnerable to entry from other providers, and others to the argument that their value has not been demonstrated.

On the other hand, demand for some of the core activities of the hospital remains high and past experience suggests that advances in medical technology will continue to produce new forms of service. Most of the emphasis in recent debates on the scope for transfer has emphasised the possibilities of mode substitution, while ignoring the long-established tendency for the demand for hospital-based services to grow through the development of new services. In most industries, dominant suppliers begin at some stage to lose custom to other providers: the successful ones respond by developing new services or products. In a sense that is what has happened to the acute hospital during the 1980s. Care outside the hospital has steadily increased in importance, but the hospital itself has continued to develop new 'lines of business', such as the anti-coagulants, and reduce the costs to the patient and the NHS of some existing ones by, for example, reducing lengths of stay.

In other words, demand for hospital services is not bottomless, even in a health service which is free at the point of access. Rather, the pool of demand is being constantly replenished.

Martin and Smith (1995) have found that the length of waiting lists does respond to extra expenditure, but the nature of their evidence, a cross-section comparison between different parts of the country, does not bear on the potential for 'topping up'. Furthermore, demand for the emergency facilities of the acute hospital continues to grow, at least in some areas. That, in itself, should give pause to those who assume that the balance of care will inevitably switch away from the hospital.

Moreover, many parts of the country do not enjoy the best pattern of care affordable within current levels of funding. In these instances, of which cancer care is perhaps the best example, there is scope recognised in the recent report of the Expert Advisory Group on Cancer Services (Department of Health, 1994) for expansion of services in at least those parts of the country where services are poor to bring them up to the level obtained in the rest of the UK.

The significance of these conclusions for the themes of this report – the scope and scale of hospitals – is not easy to assess. Many of the areas of potential substitution apply to virtually all hospital providers, whatever their scale or scope; changes in the pattern of care of even the most specialised may be feasible, eg in the area of post-operative support. Equally, pressure to eliminate procedures which are not effective applies across the board. While changes in demography and in the pattern of disease may seem to favour either smaller hospitals or intermediate institutions, we have argued against drawing that conclusion. Other factors, eg the trends observed in emergency care, may favour larger units which might be better able to cope with peaks and troughs and provide the full range of facilities required. But whether that is so depends critically on the way that the supply of hospital services is likely to change and it is to that we turn in the following chapter.

CHAPTER 9

The supply of hospital services

This chapter is concerned primarily with two questions:

- will developments in the supply of hospital services tend to make those services, however delivered, more attractive to purchasers through lowering their costs, improving quality or in other ways?
- how will these developments influence the pattern of provision of hospital services: will they encourage dispersal or concentration of services by reducing or increasing cost thresholds or by emphasising or countering the advantages of scale and scope?

First, however, we consider how the supply of hospital services has been changing in recent years.

9.1 The changing hospital

Ever since the foundation of the NHS, acute hospitals have been closing beds, reducing lengths of stay and, as they have been treating more patients, increasing their levels of bed utilisation. This picture holds for hospital activity as a whole, at the level of specialty and also for individual procedures: see Tables 9.1, 9.2 and 9.3.

These changes have been effected in the face of demographic trends that have worked against them. Not only are older people admitted more often, but they also stay longer when they are admitted. Analysis by Harrison and Boyle (1993) showed that, during the 1980s, the impact of

Table 9.1 Average length of stay (days), ordinary admissions, non-psychiatric hospitals: England

	1981	1992/93
Non-surgical acute	10.2	6.3
Surgical acute	7.5	4.8
Geriatrics	66.1	23.5
Maternity	5.5	2.9

Source: Department of Health Statistical Bulletins

Table 9.2 Average length of stay: selected conditions

	1981		1993	
	Males	Females	Males	Females
All	11.6	16.6	7.9	12.2
Infectious diseases	13.9	12.9	6.5	7.9
Malignant neoplasms	13.4	14.4	9.4	10.2
Benign neoplasms	7.3	8.1	5.1	6.1
Diseases of nervous system	37.1	54.4	20.3	33.9
Diseases of eye	8.6	9.4	3.3	4.0
Diseases of ear	4.1	4.5	2.2	2.4
Heart disease	13.7	30.6	7.0	12.0
Cerebrovascular disease	48.3	85.5	41.1	67.8
Diseases of respiratory system	14.6	28.4	10.9	18.9
Diseases of digestive system	7.9	10.2	4.8	6.3

Source: Scottish Health Statistics

Table 9.3 Bed utilisation: acute cases per bed, per year

1959	1969	1979	1993/94
14.7	19.7	23.4	55.4

Source: Health and Personal Social Statistics

growth in the numbers of very elderly people using hospital was more than countered by the increasing rate of throughput:

> ... if lengths of stay had not fallen within each age group, but all other changes had taken place as in fact they did, the average would have risen by nearly two days. In fact, the average in 1990 was 9.5 days. Thus had not length of stay fallen in each group as it did, the average would have been some 59 per cent greater than it actually is. Thus the overall reduction of stay from 1980 to 1990 has been 28 per cent but this is a result of two opposing effects: the change in age structure and discharge rates pushing the average up and the effect of clinical and managerial changes pushing it down.

Their analysis also suggested that change in the composition of activity, ie the balance of work between specialties also had little effect on average lengths of stay.

While inpatient stays have been falling, the volume of day care has increased. The volume of cases treated on a day basis rose by over 150 per cent during the 1980s, for all age groups and across most surgical specialties. To some unknown extent, however, the rise in day case numbers reflects a reclassification of work, eg from outpatient to day inpatient and to better recording. This effect is likely to have been stimulated by government attempts to encourage day care but there is no way of saying by how much.

The combination of shorter stays and higher proportions of day surgery means that the number of bed days, ie overnight stays, has risen much less fast than the number of patients treated. Between 1981 and 1991, the number of inpatient days in English acute hospitals declined from just under 49 million to just under 46 million. The role of the hospital in England as an inpatient institution is now in decline.

All the changes described here, apart from the rapid increase in day surgery, are of long standing; taken together, however, they have now reached a point where the nature of the acute hospital is being transformed. The typical currency for describing the size of the hospital, the staffed bed, is now outmoded. More significantly, as the balance of inpatient activity has moved heavily towards the provision of emergency care, the management issues posed by the variable nature of that demand will increase.

Although bed numbers in geriatric and acute specialties have fallen from 200,000 in 1981 to 147,000 in 1993/94, in all other ways that we can measure, hospitals absorb more resources than ever before. As noted in Chapter 1, the total number of doctors working in hospitals has risen, in absolute terms and as a proportion of total medical labour force. Their skills are increasingly specialised. There are no data which allow the pattern of work actually done by hospital doctors to be measured and hence the extent to which they specialise in particular areas of clinical activity. Although most doctors continue to class themselves as generalist, the proportion which do has fallen: see Table 9.4. With two exceptions, growth in the numbers of specialists was higher than the numbers assigned to either general medicine or general surgery. These figures almost certainly understate the trend towards greater specialisation in part because generalists in practice specialise and in part because specialists themselves specialise within sub-specialties.

Even in relatively small specialties such as ophthalmology or plastic surgery, sub-specialties are developing, based on particular procedures, but changes of this kind are not reflected in the available figures.

Table 9.4 Hospital medical workforce by specialty

	(Selected Categories)		
	1981	1992	Change
			%
General Medicine	3,989	4,796	120
Rheumatology	432	435	101
Chest	428	299	70
Dermatology	368	442	120
Cardiology	291	515	177
Geriatrics	1,615	1,948	121
Ophthalmology	993	1,180	114
Paediatrics	1,723	2,537	147
General Surgery	3,456	3,561	103
ENT	886	1,043	117
Trauma/Orthopaedic	1,843	2,381	129
Plastics	198	320	162
Cardio-Thoracic	310	413	133
Neurosurgery	228	256	112
Obstetrics/Gynaecology	2,480	3,017	122

Source: Health and Personal Social Services Statistics for England: figures are whole time equivalents

The number of nurses employed in hospitals has not changed much in recent years, falling from 327,000 in 1981 to 313,000 in 1992. That is what we would expect, given the reduction in inpatient care. The number of technicians, however, has increased rapidly, rising from just under 14,000 in 1981 to 29,000 in 1991.

While we can present some information relating to human resources, it is less easy to describe the availability of capital equipment. Until recently, there were no records of the physical assets used by hospitals. Although, as a result of the reforms introduced through the NHS and Community Care Act 1990, all providers have to set up asset registers, no published data are available for the period before the Act came into force. While it is commonly accepted that hospitals have more equipment at their disposal now than 10 or more years ago, just how much more is hard to demonstrate. In its 1994 public expenditure report, the House of Commons Health Select Committee published figures for the current value of the capital stock used within the NHS as a whole but similar figures are not available for the period before the introduction of the NHS and Community Care Act (1990).

Leaving capital assets to one side, the physical productivity of the hospital has risen. Whatever measure is used, labour or bed productivity, hospitals have improved their performance. According to Cutler (1993), the efficiency with which human resources were used grew by a little under two per cent per annum between 1979/80 and 1990/91. These figures do not attempt to identify any cost shifting that might have occurred to general practitioners or to community nursing staff as a consequence of shorter lengths of stay. Although both GPs and nursing staff working outside hospitals believe that cost-shifting has occurred, it is not possible to demonstrate it in numerical terms. Nor it is possible, as already pointed out, for changes in the use of capital resources to be taken into account. With these qualifications, the picture that emerges is of a hospital system expanding in terms of activity, using more highly trained staff and doing more with those resources.

9.2 Technology

The changes in hospital services described above have been largely driven by changes in medical technology which have strengthened the role of the hospital by increasing the range of what it can do and reducing the cost of some procedures. In addition, technological development in support services, from information handling to meal preparation, has also allowed costs to be reduced and thereby improved the overall competitiveness of the hospital.

Further implementation of existing technology will have a major impact on hospital services. The scope for increased use of day surgery is apparent from reports by the Audit Commission (refs) and the Government's own Day Surgery Task Force (NHS Management Executive, 1993). In addition, minimally invasive techniques look set to transform the way that some, if not most, surgery is carried out and the skills needed to perform it. *Minimal Access Surgery* (1994) (generally known as the Cushieri Report) suggests that in 10 years' time, 70 per cent of surgical operations will be carried out in this way, but adds:

> *The overall impact on NHS costs (both hospital and community) may not be significant but there are substantial gains for patients in the quality and acceptability of the care they receive and for the Exchequer in reduced sickness and other benefits. (p 22)*

Although recently some reservations have been expressed, particularly on the need for training and on the overall economics of the new procedures, on balance they appear likely to be more widely adopted than they are now. If so, that is likely to strengthen the position of the acute general hospital since most procedures require the back-up resources likely to be found there, even if the procedures themselves, like some day surgery units, are actually carried out in adjacent but separate facilities. Furthermore, as the new techniques have less impact on the patient, they should allow intervention rates to rise, particularly for the elderly. In the words of a recent review (Schwartz 1994):

> . . . it is likely that further advances in surgery that reduce risk and pain (such as laparoscopy and arthroscopy) will open the door to many more surgical procedures. Patients with less severe illnesses and those for whom traditional surgical procedures pose an excessive risk will become suitable candidates for new therapies (p 78).

Developments in those areas of surgical techniques are relatively easy to forecast and their impact relatively easy to envisage even if the rate of change and the full extent of their impact remain unclear. They will reduce bed requirements, but that in itself will not change the role of the hospital. Whether they alter the balance between different hospital configurations depends critically on whether the new techniques can, once training is on a proper footing, be used safely and effectively on most hospital sites.

Over and above the wider application of existing techniques, a large number of new developments are on the horizon or even within sight. Some examples taken from Banta's (1990) wide-ranging review of the scope for new treatment methods are:

- organ transplantation, including artificial animal organs and the use of inbuilt micro computers to aid drug release
- biotechnology leading to improved monitoring procedures and more specific drug, vaccine and hormone treatments, including artificial blood cells
- genetic diagnosis and therapy, leading to better and earlier diagnoses or the elimination of certain categories of disease.

Some, such as gene therapy, might transform the workload of the hospital; others, such as artificial organs, would accentuate trends already present. The scope for innovation extends to diagnostics as well as treatment: see Box 9.1.

The key question is whether further advances in medical technology will promote further interdependence or the opposite by creating techniques which promote separability. It appears particularly hard to come to a clear view as to which effect will dominate. On the one hand, it seems reasonable to assume that medical knowledge will continue to develop and that the scope for specialisation will increase across the whole clinical labour force. Most specialties appear to assume that further specialisation is either desirable or inevitable or both and that would seem to work in favour of larger clusters than is typical now. Rees (1995) argues that 'the inexorable growth of specialism will continue'. On the other hand, some developments allow generalists be it the GP, nurse or even the patient, to administer treatment safely which was once the preserve of specialists. Furthermore, specialists are developing within nursing or technical support who can reduce the need for larger clusters of medical staff.

As things stand, the changes Schwartz foresees – see Box 9.1 – will tend to strengthen the role of the hospital, the current location for more expensive equipment. However, there have been developments which point the other way which combine both new technology and new forms of economic organisations. As Stilwell (1993) has shown in relation to pathology services, the economics of laboratory operation are now such that concentration of activity is not essential to economical provision. A number of different provision models are available, which can be adapted to different sizes of hospital. One such model is the free-standing diagnostic centre which is available to hospitals of all sizes and hence all sizes of unit to enjoy whatever scale economies exist and of course to other, now hospital providers as well. Similarly, digitalisation of imaging results allows them to be rapidly available to anyone connected to the appropriate network. Developments such as those again demonstrate how forces making for concentration and dispersal can co-exist..

The same is true of information technology. As far as information technology itself goes, there appears to be every reason to expect that costs will come down and potential performance go up. This potential may be exploited in a number of ways:

- more large-scale communications networks
- larger databases with easier access
- improved capacity for epidemiological analysis and clinical decision-making
- better information for patients
- new ways of training doctors.

These developments cut in more than one way. Some will provide benefits wherever care is delivered. Some will strengthen the position of large providers by improving their powers of analysis and hence the ability both to understand the market they serve and their own internal operation.

Box 9.1: Improvements in diagnostics

■ Improvements in computed tomography (CT) scanning and magnetic resonance imaging (MRI) will greatly enhance the diagnostic power of these devices and expand the volume of scanning procedures. Scanning of the heart is a dramatic exercise. The moving heart has previously defied accurate definition by CT scans and MRI, but new techniques will soon allow the motion of the heart to be 'frozen' so that sharp images can be obtained. With refinements in these methods, the detection of even the early stages of coronary artery disease will be possible.

■ Advances in MRI, PET scanning, and magnetoencephalography also will provide new tools for evaluating mental illness and other brain disorders and for assessing the effectiveness of treatment.

■ Two imaging techniques that are nearing clinical application promise significant advances in diagnostic capabilities. The first, coherence interferometry, provides detailed images of the top few millimetres of a given organ by capturing the faint light that is reflected off the tissue. Preliminary studies suggest that the degree of detail can come close to that which is now obtained with stained histologic tissue sections. Such 'optical biopsies' will open a wide range of diagnostic possibilities for organs whose surfaces are readily accessible, such as the eye, colon, and coronary arteries. The technique should be particularly useful in the diagnosis and management of eye disorders such as glaucoma and retinal disease. A second technique, new and sophisticated methods of transillumination, promises to add significantly to diagnostic capabilities by its ability to recognise subtle tissue abnormalities. Imaging of brain bleeding, brain tumors, and oxygen deficits in the brain are already in clinical trials. Transillumination also promises to be useful in imaging the breast, prostate, and testicles and to identify structures within cells (for example, nuclei and mitochondria).

■ In the more distant future lie the medical applications of 'virtual reality'. Work now in progress suggests that it will be practical to use virtual reality techniques to obtain a precise spatial perspective on internal body organs. High-speed computers in combination with ultrasound will be used to create a 'virtual hole' in the patient's body that will display a given organ in three dimensions. By looking into an ultrasound 'peephole', surgeons will be able, for example, to perform amniocentesis and many types of biopsies with great precision. This method also will create three-dimensional images for the surgeon working inside an organ. When used preoperatively, the virtual reality technique will enable the surgeon to plan operative surgery with simulated body structures.

Source: Schwartz (1994)

In general, however, developments in this area appear to favour dispersed modes of delivering care since they reduce the need for physical transfer of information or people. Not only can the results of tests be transferred electronically, but expertise can be consulted 'at a distance', either through particular individuals, thereby allowing quality to be supervised without actually bringing the skilled staff to one place, or in the more abstract sense, of allowing ready access through appropriate organised data banks or expert systems, to the knowledge which has accumulated worldwide in whatever area needs to be consulted. In the UK and elsewhere, a small number of services using tele-medicine operate on a quasi-experimental basis. For example, the Riverside Community Trust in Central London operate a minor injuries unit which is linked to a major accident and emergency department in another part of the UK. However, while developments such as this which allow a small-scale facility safely to extend the range of work it can take on, they also strengthen those existing centres whose expertise is consulted, allowing them to serve much larger areas than their 'own' districts. In other words, they simultaneously promote centralisation and decentralisation.

Overall, the likely impact of developments in information technology remains hard to define in terms of specific effects, since so many new possibilities are opening up, and the costs of computing power continue to decline. The only safe conclusion appears to be that developments are loosening some of the connections that have promoted clustering of activities in hospitals in the past, but they do not point clearly to any one set of alternative clusters. A more speculative but reasonable conclusion would be their main impact will be on what was termed in Chapter 3 the 'routing process', by making it easier for professionals working outside the hospital to make clinical decisions.

In other words, technological development in the broad sense considered here is working to create more delivery options and in that sense it undermines the existing pattern of provision. Vague though that conclusion is, it serves to underline one of the main points made in Chapter 4, that the balance between hospitals and other providers should be seen as fluid; there will be gains here and losses there, but no 'steady state'. As Banta (1993) in a wide-ranging review of medical technology puts it:

> For the future, the tension between centralisation and decentralisations seem likely to grow. (p36)

What should the hospital planner make of these conclusions? Perhaps the central point is that if the scope for new forms of care delivery is expanding, there is no reason to expect that one best solution will emerge. It therefore does not make sense to attempt to forecast where the balance will be, in part because a variety of 'solutions' may be sensible, depending on local circumstances, in part because the outcome will depend on the incentives facing each of the many actors in the health care system and their scope for independent action. This is not a comfortable conclusion, emphasising as it does the uncertainties that lie ahead. It argues against blueprint planning in favour of flexible solutions. And in health care delivery, flexible solutions are not always easy to define.

9.3 Human resources

There will inevitably be disagreement about the speed at which technological developments will actually take place and their likely impact. But even those developments which can be foreseen may transform the way hospital work is organised. Minimal access techniques, for example, threaten the traditional role of the surgeon. Warner *et al* (1994) raise the question whether:

> *[the] stance of specialists in the face of this innovation is not in the best public interest but is protectionist and monopolistic. Is there scope for developing a less fully trained endoscopist who can be as technically proficient at a lower overall cost....Already in some countries there has been a lively debate about whether there should be a separate specialty for endoscopists. (p 74)*

Similarly, Wickham (1993) suggests that surgeons 'are going to have to accept the changing status of being only one member of a group of interventionalists' and indeed have a declining role:

> *It may well be that organ specific physicians will after diagnosis direct the patient to the most efficient 'sub-contractor interventionalist'. (p 13)*

In these ways, possible changes in the technology used to provide hospital services could transform the way that medical and other human resources are used within the hospital. However, changes in the way that hospital staff, particularly medical staff, are organised are under-way for an entirely different set of reasons.

For some time, Government policy has been directed at raising the proportion of consultant level staff as an essential step towards improving the quality of care. The immediate stimulus to this was a report by the Social Services Committee of the House of Commons on Medical

Education (House of Commons, 1981) which argued for the primacy of medical care over the career and training needs of doctors. It recommended an increase in the ratio of consultant to training posts in most hospitals. Progress in implementing that proved slow, but in 1987 the health departments and the professions published *Hospital Medical Staffing: Achieving a Balance* (Department of Health, 1987), designed to make progress easier.

More recently, two further developments have begun to undermine existing staffing arrangements.

- the Government's intention to reduce junior doctors' hours which means that cover will have to be provided by senior staff
- the changes in medical education consequent on harmonising with the European Community.

These changes, combined with the scope for innovation now offered to trusts, will mean that - new staffing patterns for hospital services and complementary community-based services can and must emerge.

Some of the impacts are fairly easy to identify. A reduction in junior doctors hours reduces the effective number available, and makes it impossible for them to ensure 24-hour medical cover in the way they do now. The greater commitment of consultant time to formal training of junior staff, which changes to medical education require, will have the same effect. This will create stronger pressures in the direction of a greater concentration of skills, particularly in the specialties where 24-hour emergency cover is required. If the lessons of CEPOD cited in Chapter 5 come to be accepted, then purchasers may insist on more extensive consultant on-site cover than is usual now.

The implications are potentially far-reaching. In the case of the medical specialities, who are largely responsible for emergency admissions, it seems plausible to assume that the changes will create pressures for greater specialisation within general medicine, ie that as consultants take over more direct responsibility for care, they will seek to maintain their special interests in particular categories of patient. If they do so, then that combined with the quality requirement of 24-hour cover will lead to greater concentrations of experienced physicians. Thus the overall effect seems likely to reinforce the arguments set out above for concentrating medical resources for these services, and in this way to further increase the size of the minimum viable unit, particularly in relation to emergency care.

The scale of this effect depends critically on the work schedules that trusts are able to negotiate with their consultants, the strength of the Government's commitment to reducing junior doctors' hours and also on the scope for developing new skill mixes, involving other clinical staff. Only a very small number of hospitals are currently operating on a 24-hour consultant cover basis and then only in some non-medical specialties, so there is little experience to go on.

The nature of the issues and the current lack of agreement about them are brought out in a discussion document from the British Paediatric Association, *Hospital Paediatric Medical Staffing*(1991). The document is quite frank about the difficulties the Association faced in coming to a view about the implication of the change in hours and the need to preserve cover not only within paediatrics but also in respect of maternity, accident and emergencies and for surgical specialties treating children. It records that there is no agreement on the question of the minimum size of a children's service to ensure quality and safety, irrespective of staffing or economic considerations. But the analysis presented of the impact of reduction in junior doctors' hours suggests that some small units would have to close to maintain cover with existing staffing levels. It also points out that further amalgamations where there is currently more than one hospital in any area would also make it possible to maintain standards within existing staffing limits.

Here, the key issue is how best to deploy a skilled labour force, the numbers of which are deemed to be effectively fixed in the short run. Even though the small unit may be viable in itself, a case may be made for concentrating staff in the interests of the service as a whole, since experienced staff will see more patients in a larger centre. The assumption critical to this conclusion, commonly made in discussions of the medical workforce is that the supply of trained staff is fixed in the short and the medium term. How true this is, and how long it will remain so, is rarely questioned: in some specialties recruitment of non-British nationals has proved feasible, though usually of doctors still undergoing training.

However, while these developments reinforce the arguments for concentrating services, other developments point the other way. As trusts learn how to effectively exploit the greater freedom they enjoy to set their own contracts, it will be much easier to staff innovative services, including medical services for which community trusts are responsible, for example, by increasing the number of community-based consultants in specialties such as paediatrics and geriatrics or, as the British Paediatric Association point out in the discussion document referred to above, developing new ways of service delivery involving hospital out-reach. Moreover, much more radical developments in the market for medical manpower are becoming feasible. Up to now, the medical labour market has been characterised by restriction and lack of innovation. As Maynard and Walker (1993) have pointed out:

No other sector has tenure ... or an absence of challenge or payments systems quite like that enjoyed by NHS doctors. (p 26)

This may be about to alter. The changes impelled by the European Community together with the changes already mentioned will reduce the hold of the Royal Colleges over medical appointments and staffing structures. Also relevant is a recent successful appeal by a non-EU doctor with extensive work experience in this country against the BMA against refusal of registration. As a result, the market for medical personnel will become much more like a normal labour market, allowing new forms of service delivery to be established. It will be much easier, for example, to develop free-standing facilities and to move staff to facilities rather than patients. Provided that functions are clinically and economically separable, it should prove easier than it has been up to now to staff them satisfactorily.

At the moment, a major obstacle to innovation in staffing structures lies in the link between service provision and training. Hospitals which do not provide what the Royal Colleges consider the right pattern of work find it hard to recruit and retain medical staff: hospitals not providing the 'right' mix of work find recruitment difficult. However, the link between medical training and hospital structure is being eroded. One of the central arguments for retaining large general hospitals is the need to provide for the training of doctors. Any dispersal would make it harder for them to see a wide cross-section of cases. Already, however, the changes described above in the way that hospitals function are leading to changes in the way that medical education is provided, away from concentration on the teaching hospital site towards the notion of the teaching district. It seems likely as the shift to community-based physicians increases that it will have to change further.

Training apart, there is scope for changing the way that doctors work within hospitals. The Audit Commission's report on the work of hospital doctors *The Doctor's Tale* (1995) makes a series of recommendations designed to make hospitals both more efficient and more flexible institutions, (the title being chosen to reflect the archaic practices they found on some hospital sites):

Doctors should be deployed more efficiently to meet both service and training needs:

- *junior doctors' basic working hours should be allocated more flexibly across the day;*
- *shift and partial-shift systems should be encouraged because they offer advantages to both patients and doctors;*
- *protected time for handover between shifts and rotas is needed to ensure continuity of patient care;*
- *the number of tiers of staff providing emergency cover should be reduced if the demand is not sufficient for the current number; and*
- *where appropriate, specialties should also be combined to provide emergency cover (p 35).*

As this analysis makes clear, the way that doctors, particularly senior ones work, can and must change. By how much depends in part on the roles of their colleagues in other professions.

Up to now, it has been the organisation of medical staff as well as their training and research requirements which has dominated thinking about the hospital: the developments described so far in this section represent a continuation of that mode of thinking. However, changes within nursing bear on the competitive position of the hospital, but in conflicting ways. Overall, under the influence of Project 2000, the trend is for nurses to be more highly qualified. That leads in at least two directions: first, it increases the opportunities for nurse/doctor substitution within the hospital, and makes new ways of service delivery clinically feasible. Second, it increases the scope for dispersing expertise away from the hospital, through the development of specialist nurses working in intermediate institutions or giving domiciliary care.

Such opportunities are already apparent. It is becoming increasingly common to find specialist nurses carrying out tasks which either replace doctors, particularly junior ones, or complement generalist physicians with their specialist knowledge, inside and outside the hospital. One example from inside the hospital is the use of a specialist asthma nurse alongside a general physician. The use of specialist nurses in this way allows blends of general and specialist expertise to be available that would be much more expensive using medical staff alone. The effect is to alter the quality/cost threshold to the extent that this is dominated by the need to concentrate medical staff.

The scope for change can be illustrated by changes made at the John Radcliffe Hospital in Oxford. In this case, the nature of the working relationship between professional groups is being transformed from one of hierarchy to partnership, a context which makes shifts of role easier to accomplish.

The John Radcliffe team report (personal communication) that:

> *There is a demand to change the culture of care. In our experiment we have moved from the traditional doctor led system to team based disciplinary care. We are steadily moving to a system where the patient is managed by the nurse in a true primary nurse role. This requires a higher skill mix in nursing staff (many being graduate nurses). Ultimately we envisage the patient having their medical care prescribed by the surgeon, rehabilitation prescribed by the physiotherapist and their home support prescribed by the occupational therapist with the primary nurse, as the only holder of the intimate knowledge of the patient's requirements, managing each 24 hour period of the patient's care, prioritising the requests. Discharge planning will be a nurse/physiotherapy function working within the surgical management plan.*

The changes introduced there have involved substantial re-organisation of working schedules for all the grades of staff involved. Consultants will have a lower proportion of personal time in their new schedule but a much higher involvement with patients. On-call time for all staff is reduced. In return, substantial benefits are claimed:

> *The manpower provision required to provide such a service is significantly more. Increased efficiency by senior input not only reduces the length of stay, reduces complications, and meets patients and purchasers expectations. In trauma the initial assessment, diagnosis and surgery is the critical part of care and consultants involvement at this time is undoubtedly cost effective. Problems cost money in terms of increased length of stay, cost of corrective surgery and expensive drugs.*

How large the scope for substitution between different professional groups or for redefining the role of those groups is hard to establish. Some studies suggest a great deal; analysis with the Northern General Hospital Trust in Sheffield (Cohen, 1993) found that substantial areas of work normally carried out by junior doctors could be carried out successfully by specially trained support workers.

Another study in the Trent region (Read and Gravin, 1994) concluded that nursing posts designed primarily to reduce the workload of doctors in training had succeeded in doing so, and that patient care had also improved. McKee and Black (1991) cite a number of studies suggesting that much of the hospital doctor's workload, particularly the junior doctors', has no medical content and hence can be done by others. Similarly, Dowling *et al* (1995) report the successful substitution of doctors by nurses in a number of roles. In general, however (Richardson and Maynard, 1995), it is hard to demonstrate the overall net benefits of this kind of substitution, as few rigorous studies exist of the combined economies and clinical benefits of using different skill-mixes.

Outside the hospital, specialist nurses may reduce the need for hospital referral. In respect of care for the mentally ill, the number of community psychiatric nurses has been rising rapidly in recent years, though from a very low base. Frequently, they receive referrals directly from GPs, thus cutting out the link via the hospital based consultant. In the case of care for children, in a number of areas specialist paediatric nurses are enabling care to be switched from the hospital to the home. More generally, the Government announced in November 1993 that it proposed to introduce community nurse prescribing for a limited range of drugs on a trial basis.

In the US, the Office of Technology Assessment has estimated that advanced practice nurses can meet the needs of 50–90 per cent of patients receiving care outside the hospital. Aitken and Sage (1993) cite this and other evidence to suggest that nurses can directly substitute for hospital doctors – 65 per cent of all anaesthetics administered in the US are the responsibility of nurses – or indirectly through the provision of ambulatory (ie community- or home-based) options. There, as in the UK, however, there are substantial barriers to change arising from traditional definitions of professional roles. The difference now perhaps is that the pressures on the medical workforce arising from the factors discussed here are such that the barriers will have to go. The 1995 Report of the Medical Workforce Standing Advisory Committee concluded that:

9.8 *A number of Trusts are developing new and diverse healthcare roles. These roles have frequently been established on an ad hoc basis, often to meet a local staffing need. Some have been running successfully for several years and are to continue and expand, others are less certain of a future. There has been proliferation and hybridization of the original schemes resulting from a growing awareness of their usefulness and success. There are several overlapping categories in the development of new clinical roles: substitution of one professional group by another; extension or expansion of work already done by an established occupational group; and the evolution of new occupational groups with differing training backgrounds...*

9.9 *Many of the present schemes involve an extended role for nurses, the largest but by no means only professional group, which might change its working practices.*

Other groups – scientific staff, physiotherapists, technicians, medical secretaries, ward clerks – have the potential to expand their role. There is now widespread acceptance that many tasks which are currently performed by medical staff could be undertaken effectively by other professional groups. Whilst it is clearly undesirable to have highly trained and relatively expensive medical staff engaged on inappropriate tasks, changing the skill mix is also an opportunity to increase the scope, challenge and interest of other staff.

9.10 Various professions are looking at ways in which they might accommodate the changes in the health service within and around their own disciplines. For example, the Royal College of Radiologists recently advised its Fellows to re-examine the working relationships of physicians and other professionals working in clinical radiology and clinical oncology, outlining extended roles in a number of areas such as ultrasound scanning, intravenous injections, the organisation of clinical trials and research. (p59)

A consequence, as Moss and McNichol argue (1995), is that new models of organisation are required:

Consultants should not expect or be expected to do three jobs at once. Clinical specialists need to focus on assuring the delivery of effective and appropriate care to the population. Their role as experts in emergency care may need to be separated from their role as specialists to a population. Those who train or manage should be trained to do so and given the time to do these things properly.

The Calman Committee's proposals look daunting. But doctors in training, who, with nurses, have absorbed most of the pressures of the relentless increase in the pace of delivering care, need a better deal. If this is to be achieved then changes in the organisation of health care professionals are essential. Getting the roles of senior specialists sorted out must be part of a bigger rethink of the best way to deliver health care. The health service needs to start considering and trying alternative models of organisation now – remembering that after the implementation of the Calman recommendations the number of trained and certified specialists will increase as the training will be shorter. The changes needed may be painful. But unless the service faces up to the need to restructure and reorganise, everyone, especially patients, will be losers. (p 928)

The implications of this could be very far-reaching, since they suggest that some of the glue that currently binds the various functions of the hospital together may have to be dissolved. Similarly, though in a more limited sphere, the 1995 Report of the Medical Workforce Standing Advisory Committee suggests that:

> *10.10 Implementation of the Calman Report will provide a more intensive and structured training for junior doctors and may require some consultants to spend more of their time on teaching and supervision of training. It is possible that some individuals and possibly whole Trusts, might in future opt out of training junior doctors altogether. The net effect on consultants' clinical time will not be clear for some years.*

The conclusion to be drawn from this discussion of manpower is similar to that on technology, that the changes that can be anticipated tend to create opportunities for new forms of care delivery. That may tend to work against the hospital as presently structured, but agile management will be able to exploit the new opportunities to reduce costs and offer more attractive services. Thus the prospect is one of continuous change in the way that hospitals are staffed and organised. But from the viewpoint of their competitiveness it is the impact on their cost of provision which counts: we turn to this next.

9.4 Cost levels

The performance of UK hospitals during the 1980s demonstrated a sustained ability to make better use of both physical assets and manpower. There seems no reason why performance in these senses should not continue to improve, for several reasons:

- the technical impulses underlying them are far from exhausted and indeed, as we saw in the earlier paragraphs, there is clear expectation of further improvement in surgical technique
- the scope for cost reduction in non-clinical areas has been demonstrated by a series of reports by their external auditors, the Audit Commission and the National Audit Office
- the scope for getting better skill mix should be greater in view of the changes described in the previous section
- the pressures to make improvements and hence to force change through are likely to grow rather than diminish.

The hard question is: what is the likely scale of cost reduction? Claims that hospital costs can be reduced by large amounts are now commonplace. Drawing on audit reports and other sources, a group of senior doctors in Wales (Roberts, 1995) suggested a figure of 20 per cent. Given that so many elements are involved ranging from surgical technique to cleaning costs, no specific figures can be more than speculative since the ramifications of change can be complex. New surgical techniques appear to promise lower costs, but it is hard to demonstrate by how much. In respect of non-invasive surgery, the Brunel study already drawn on

(Sculpher, 1993) emphasises that it is not yet possible to identify the full cost implications of the introduction of these techniques. In particular:

- it is not easy to identify the base-line, given the rapid introduction of day surgery based on conventional techniques
- some minimal access techniques increase demands on hospital resources
- although initial hospitalisation is normally reduced, in some cases return visits have proved higher than with traditional techniques.

Outside the hospital, minimal access surgery offers benefits in terms of shorter recovery periods and, probably, less home-delivered care and while these benefits do not accrue to the provider of hospital services they should appeal to purchasers who are able to take a view across the health care sector as a whole. At present, the knowledge needed to evaluate all the consequences taken together is not available.

The evidence cited by Roberts and his colleagues has been derived from studies of current practice by the Audit Commission and others. But the previous sections of this chapter have suggested that the status quo will not continue, particularly in the areas of human resources. However, given the limited experience available and the tentative nature of some of the experimental staffing methods mentioned above, it is hard to form a view of the potential impact on costs: indeed, the main impact of the changes made at the John Radcliffe should be on quality rather than costs, although as noted cost savings were expected in some areas. Furthermore, particularly in respect of emergency care, pressure to raise quality in the light of the failings identified in Chapter 5 may well work the other way, if that means higher levels of experienced medical staff being available at all times In respect of elective work, the scope for cost reduction seems clearer, but if the reservations expressed by Sculpher are correct, then here too quality may take precedence over cost reduction. Thus, although the Government via purchasers continues to press for more activity from the same or fewer financial resources, while at the same time pressing, through the *Patient's Charter* standards, for higher levels of service, it has no means at its disposal of estimating whether it can simultaneously achieve these objectives and improve clinical outcomes through the introduction of new methods of treatment. It is, moreover, hard to discern whether it will prove easier to achieve lower costs/higher quality in some hospital configurations than others. Cost factors may tilt the balance in respect of emergency care in favour of greater concentration of activity. But the scope for skill substitution combined with developments in information technology could for some part of the workload tilt the balance back echoing once again Banta's conclusion on the impact of new technology.

9.5 Management structures

The essence of the general hospital, following the arguments set out in Chapter 2, lies in the way it brings together large numbers of professionals who provide services and carry out functions which, on a day-to-day basis, are often unrelated. The success of the hospital as an institution depends in large part on how well the various professionals perform their respective functions and inter-relate when they have to, which may be rarely, or very frequently.

During the 1980s, the introduction of general management was perhaps the single most important change in the management of UK hospitals. It was introduced because, in the Government's view, the existing management structures failed to ensure that common interests were properly protected and furthered by the so-called consensus management system.

This change in management technology has been generally regarded as successful, although in the nature of things that is hard to prove. Other innovations such as clinical budgeting appear to have had little impact on hospital activity. The creation of trusts has led to further innovation, eg through appointment of clinical directors, but so far change has been fairly small. Research carried out at the Institute for Manpower Studies in the first two years of the 'new' NHS discovered that most trusts were sticking to pay and manning structures with which they were already familiar, but that may be about to change, in the light of Government pressure on trusts to set up their own bargaining arrangements.

The potential for further change is considerable. In the past, medical staffing structure has been dominated by the concept of the clinical firm and the departmental hierarchical structure going with it. These arguments reflect the way hospitals developed as far back as the last century and the close links between hospital structure and teaching. The Audit Commission's report (1995) suggests that new forms of management structure will be required which, among other things, will loosen the ties between senior and junior doctors, making the latter – as indeed they often are already – into a general resource for the hospital as a whole. In the future, there is no reason why this should be the predominant form of organisation. The hospital may be an integrated 'command' organisation or it may be integrated through contracts. The same is true across the boundaries of the hospital as it now stands.

The hub and spoke arrangements discussed in Chapter 3 imply management structures ranging over a number of hospitals which do not arise from their overall integration. Given their novelty, it is not surprising that little evidence or even experience is available to indicate their merits and hence any estimate of their potential impact must be speculative. It seems safe to conclude, however, that there is scope for developing new structures for the supply of hospital services. These could be led from within the hospital, or from outside it through the development of community-based organisations serving a particular client group. Either way, the nature of the hospital as an institution could be transformed.

But that would not in itself mean that the hospital as a cluster of human and physical resources is similarly transformed. The forces determining geographical clusters are not identical to those determining organisational bundles. In the past, the two kinds of cluster have been closely linked. They need not be in the future.

9.6 Conclusion

As far as the scale, scope and structure of hospital provision are concerned, the factors discussed in this chapter point in different directions. New technology seems likely to promote both clustering and separability. So too do changes in the way that hospitals are staffed and organised. Within the complex pattern of change that seems likely to result, some hospitals will be threatened, particularly smaller institutions, squeezed between pressures for further clustering and concentration – reinforced by the evidence presented in Chapter 5 – and for dispersal to intermediate facilities.

But the evidence and argument presented in this chapter can be read another way: that overall the technology used by hospitals, including the organisation of staff, is becoming more flexible as boundaries between roles and professions are broken down and new forms of delivering care emerge. If so, that should offer any threatened institutions scope for competitive response and adaptation which may well allow them to survive.

Almost every aspect of the way that hospital services are provided, from the overall organisational framework to the specific intervention, seems set to change. For those responsible for running hospitals, that conclusion may at first sight seem an unwelcome one, promising as it does an agenda that may well be difficult to manage. The reverse of the coin, however, is that while new technology and other factors may threaten the hospital as it now is, other trends may enable it to strengthen its position. Within that broadly comforting conclusion, the current role of some, if not many, existing institutions may be threatened sometimes by short run forces such as shortages of particular classes of manpower. But the scope for competitive response through innovation is large and seems set to grow.

CHAPTER 10

Access: prospects and policies

Within the framework developed earlier, the value of access is one of the key determinants of hospital structure; the more important this is, the stronger the case for clustering and concentration of clinical activity. While trade-offs between quality, cost and access are inevitable, they can be modified and their impact reduced for hospital users as a whole or for those groups within the population on whom they fall most heavily. This chapter considers a range of options which are available to those responsible for planning hospital services if they wish to take access into account. We begin, however, by briefly considering the factors which might alter the nature and scale of the access issue in future years.

10.1 Travel prospects

Evidence presented in Chapter 7 suggests that some sections of the population find access to existing hospitals difficult. The question to be considered here is whether the transport sector is likely to change in ways which will reduce those difficulties.

Travel to hospital, like other health services, is predominantly carried out by car: the proportion of trips made this way has been rising, in line with trends in the transport sector as a whole. The trends of the past 30 years seem set to continue: according to Department of Transport forecasts, car ownership is expected to rise, despite the increase in congestion that implies, and use of public transport to decline. There are signs, in the recent reductions in the road programme and changes in planning policy, that the Government is beginning to consider policies designed to reduce reliance on roads and private transport. But so far there are no clear signs of policies that would actually reverse current trends and increase the availability and attractiveness of public transport.

It therefore seems reasonable to assume that the proportions travelling to hospital by car will rise. As a result, for some access will be slightly worse than it is as congestion grows; for others, ie new car-owners, it will get better. For those reliant on public transport, access will get worse in the absence of specific measures to improve it. This latter group may get smaller. Although the numbers of elderly people is rising, so are the numbers of elderly car owners, partly because incomes are higher and partly because of a 'generation' effect – more women now in their fifties learned to drive than in the earlier generation. But there will remain sizeable groups without access to cars of their own – young people, some disabled people, those on low incomes – even if car ownership as a whole continues to grow.

The relative importance of these various changes in transport will, of course, vary from place to place according to the location of hospital facilities, the transport network and the distribution of the population. In most rural areas, public transport has already virtually disappeared. In most of the larger urban centres, services remain, many serving hospitals directly. Similarly, the incidence of congestion varies from area to area. Where it is likely to worsen, in the absence of effective measures to control road use, there may be serious implications for the planning and organisation of ambulance services, eg a more dispersed siting of vehicles may be required. Furthermore, increases in journey time may tilt the balance between different forms of emergency response.

The need for travel to hospital will not remain as it is now. The changes in the workload of the hospital described in Chapter 8 are tending to alter the need to travel to it. The greater use of day surgery and shorter lengths of stay will reduce the number of people visiting inpatient departments in hospital. But as far as patients themselves are concerned, it is out- rather than inpatient visits that are important since there are vastly more of the latter. There are two reasons why travel to outpatient facilities should reduce in the future:

- most consultations and some diagnostics are separable activities and hence can be provided locally in intermediate facilities
- in some cases, steps can be taken to reduce the number of outpatient visits, particularly follow-up visits. A number of GP fundholders have used their budgets to achieve this. In Wales, a target of two follow-up visits to initial consultations has been set.

Furthermore, the impact of the *Patient's Charter* standards on waiting times in hospital outpatient departments should improve matters, for while these will not reduce the need for a journey, they will reduce the overall dislocation involved in making it. Any measures which reduce the variability of waiting times in outpatients, or of lengths of stay and discharge times, makes access easier, particularly for those who rely on public transport and who must make complicated arrangements if they are to attend hospital. Reducing uncertainty makes it easier to plan journeys and make the other arrangements associated with a hospital visit.

10.2   Policy options

The policy issues posed by access divide into three questions:

- do access difficulties pose significant costs?
- does it matter?
- what should be done if it does?

We considered the first question in Chapter 7, where our conclusion was yes, qualified by the incompleteness of the evidence. In some circumstances, poor access can create clinical risks as well as impose costs in terms of time and money and general inconvenience. While access will improve for some as a result of increasing car ownership, the groups where the volume of activity is likely to grow most – the very elderly, the chronically sick or parents with young children – are least likely to be able to use a car or afford a taxi. Thus the costs of further clustering and concentration of services may weigh heavily on those least able to bear them.

Whether that matters or not is for political – in the broad sense – judgement. In some cases, it could be argued, risks arising from poor access must be accepted as part and parcel of a particular lifestyle. People in rural areas must generally accept lower standards of access to most services, public and private. On the other hand, in some areas of public policy, there is explicit commitment to equality of access. Access to mains utilities and postal services is virtually, though not entirely, equalised and the cost differences not normally reflected in charges. In other cases such as education, policy is mixed, with free transport normally being confined to defined catchment areas. In the case of social services, transport, eg to day care facilities, is typically seen as part of the overall service.

As far as health services are concerned, policy is similarly ambivalent. Despite the NHS's long standing commitment to equality of access, the geographical aspects of inequality have typically been neglected. As Watt and Sheldon (1993) have pointed out:

> ... the health and health care of rural populations are not often seen as specific concerns by the UK's health services. (p 19)

As a result, the NHS does not have a consistent policy about whether to explicitly take rurality into account when allocating resources, on the basis of either equity or cost. Watt and Sheldon describe the variety of ways in which rurality is allowed for in different parts of the UK; these do not amount to a consistent or principled policy. The same applies to access in general. But local purchasers can take their own view as to whether to trade cost, or indeed quality, against access. If they do wish to do so, they have a number of options open to them. We divide them into five: transport options, mobile services, location options and communications and accommodation options, which we look at in turn.

Transport options

While access to ambulance services is normally restricted to those with a medical need, there is nothing to prevent health purchasers offering transport services on a wider basis. The possibilities are obvious enough and need little comment.

As public transport services of a conventional kind, ie large buses on fixed routes, have declined, a wide range of alternatives have been developed, particularly in rural areas, such as car pools, use of mail buses and voluntary car schemes. However, while these may be suited to shorter trips to a local hospital, they are less appropriate for trips over long distances to major centres of the kind which would be needed if certain types of medical and surgical work were relocated to a small number of sites. Here, dedicated provision may be required.

The scope for improving speed of access which may be important for emergency patients is largely governed by the road system. But in a few areas, helicopter transport may be of help. Helicopters operate in a few parts of the UK and if distances to major centres became longer as a result of concentration of services in trauma centres, might help to compensate. Preliminary reports on their effectiveness in London and in Cornwall by the Medical Care Research Unit at the University of Sheffield (1993) suggest that they are effective in reducing journey times in some instances and in getting patients to more appropriate settings.

In Cornwall and the Isles of Scilly, the report concludes:

> There is evidence that not only does the A/A [air ambulance] transfer patients more quickly to hospital but that they more frequently take patients to what might be more appropriate hospitals. For example, the A/A more often takes patients to major casualty departments and those with head injuries to appropriate neurosurgery facilities. The London-based service was also able to do that. It also provided more intense on-site care since they carried more junior doctors than a land-based service normally does in this country. In neither case however is outcome information yet available. (p 84)

Overall, however, services of this kind seem likely to have a very limited role by virtue of their cost and the small number of circumstances in which they offer clear-cut advantages.

Mobile services

Many services are inherently mobile since they depend on moving professionals around and not equipment. In the field of prevention, such mobility is taken for granted as it is for some of the ancillary professions such as physiotherapists. In addition, mobile operating and diagnostic facilities are technically feasible. Examples can be found in operation but they appear to be rare. A few mobile dental surgery units are in operation as well as mobile operating 'theatres' for minor procedures. The simpler end of diagnostics, such as certain screening procedures, is usually mobile but not the advanced end of the spectrum, such as CT or MRI scanners. Some advanced diagnostics are available in the US on a mobile basis but rarely in this country. In 1993, a mobile Cardiac Catheter Laboratory, the first in the country, was brought into use by St Mary's.

Location options

Chapter 4 suggested that the hierarchy of hospital provision can be seen as a strategy to improve access while maintaining quality. However, the siting of facilities can itself be made so as to improve rather than reduce access. This might mean choosing expensive sites in preference to cheaper ones. In practice, it will prove hard to find sites for whole hospitals which are accessible to both car and public transport users so the interests of some users (and staff) will have to be set against those of others. However, separable functions such as diagnostic facilities are another matter, as their space demands are much less.

To return to the retailing analogy, outpatient departments are precisely the kind of busy, high volume activities that are to be found in high streets or other accessible locations. But few NHS health facilities are to be found in such locations, even though many private health services, eg eye and dental services, are. Such a policy may seem extreme because of its inherent expense. But such sites are expensive only because they are accessible; so spending on location may save spending on other ways of improving access.

Communication options

In some cases, the need for travel can be eliminated entirely. Data transfer may reduce the need for professionals to be in close physical contact, but even the well-established technology of the telephone may have an impact on the need to travel to health facilities. A study by Wasson *et al* (1992) found that substituting telephone care for some clinics visits reduced utilisation of services on hospital sites and for some patients appeared to improve health status and reduce mortality. They concluded:

For most patients with chronic diseases, telephone care offers significant benefits: increased frequency of clinician contact, less waiting and travel time, lower cost and the possibility for improved mortality and improved function. (p 1793)

Other examples can be cited: for example, there have been experiments with provision of telephone advice from specific hospital departments. The Accident and Emergency Department at King's College Hospital operates such a service and it appears to be successful in reducing trips to the department. The Department's 1994 Activity Report records that about 70 calls are received each week – some 5 per cent of attendances – but further research is being carried out, as well as software development, to see how the service can be improved.

Other hospitals are now offering similar services. As the previous chapter indicated, the scope for 'tele-medicine' seems potentially very large (Gott, 1993) and if that is so, configurations of hospital services may be feasible and clinically satisfactory, which radically alters the need for travel. At present, tele-medicine appears to make a useful but marginal contribution to reducing the need for travel, but given the rapid pace of developments in information technology, that could quickly change.

Accommodation options

Finally, the need for travel, or the physical difficulties associated with it, can be greatly reduced by offering accommodation for overnight stays to visitors. It is common practice to offer accommodation for parents of children in hospital, but the approach can be used more generally, eg for other care groups particularly for visits to distant treatment facilities. One or two so-called patient hotels are in use for this purpose.

10.3 Conclusion

The options set out in the previous section are obvious enough. Most are technically straightforward. But because access has not been taken seriously as a general policy objective, the options have not been systematically evaluated on a service by service, area by area basis. There is little detailed analysis available of how people travel and the difficulties they face combined with an assessment of the costs of relieving those difficulties. Nor is it clear what the benefits of improving access are. The evidence cited in Chapter 8 suggested that better transport could reduce people's unwillingness to travel for particular forms of care. But the available evidence is not rich to demonstrate that effect more generally and to set its cost off against costs within the hospital system itself.

While it appears that people in general value good access, they are typically not aware of what the price – in the broad sense – of good access may be, ie a lower chance of good quality care. Indeed they have no way of forming that judgement for themselves since the volume of information about hospital performance is so limited. Any closure of hospital facilities imposes costs on those near them, for which there is no compensation mechanism, either in the direct financial sense or through the provision of transport. It is bound to be resisted.

The opportunities available for locational substitution allow services to be provided in intermediate or other units, though at unknown cost, which may improve access for these services. However, the case for provision 'closer to home' is based implicitly or explicitly on the belief that 'closer' equals 'better' though again without evidence of what may have to be sacrificed in order to get it and indeed how effective it is. Furthermore, relocation of services away from large hospitals does not in itself guarantee better access for everyone; it too requires careful analysis.

CHAPTER 11

What should be done?

This final chapter pulls the threads of the argument together to bring out the implications of the evidence and argument presented in this report for hospital planning. The central theme has been that planning hospital services involves trade-offs between quality, cost and access for whole populations or for a particular group of patients. Although much more information is available on the determinants of quality, costs and access than when the 1962 Hospital Plan was developed, knowledge is critically deficient in a number of key areas.

Perhaps the most important gap is the relationship between quality of care and hospital structure. There is some evidence suggesting that better care would result from a higher degree of concentration of activity than is currently the case in many parts of the country. But the precise nature of that relationship for each specialty or group of patients remains unclear. For some care groups, the evidence is thin: for others, where the evidence is better, the unanswered question is whether further degrees of concentration will produce benefits in terms of improved quality and/or reduced costs of provision. At the other end of the scale, it is not clear in what circumstances smaller institutions can match the quality of larger ones by modifying what they do now.

Next, the relationship between costs and different levels and composition of activity in hospitals is imperfectly understood. While it seems safe to conclude that economies of scale are not very strong, it is not clear where the thresholds are for particular activities below which costs are relatively high or quality low. Furthermore, the implications of a piecemeal withdrawal of separable functions from existing general hospitals and of substitution by other providers are not understood. This is not just a matter of accurate measurement of 'cost per case' but also rather of the overall performance of the hospital as an effective institution if that rests, to some degree, on informal as well as formal interaction between those working in it.

Finally, the importance of access, particularly the clinical costs of poor access, is not thoroughly evaluated for the full range of patients requiring the emergency facilities of the hospital. It follows that the central strategic trade-offs which lie at the heart of planning for hospitals are not precisely defined, since the differences in quality of outcome which stem from different degrees of clustering and concentration and different patterns of spatial arrangement cannot be precisely identified. Nor are those lower level trade-offs which may arise between different groups of patients as a result of choosing one pattern of care delivery rather than another.

One conclusion follows easily from this brief summary: that it would be foolish to attempt to define a blueprint for the future of the acute general hospital in the specific terms used in the 1962 Hospital Plan. Nevertheless, the overall environment – economic, political, technological – will compel change. Those responsible for thinking about the future of specific hospitals and alternatives to them must make some judgements on which to base their planning, but these will, given the prospects of continuing change, inevitably have to be tentative. Uncertainty cannot be dispelled simply by more careful analysis.

Nevertheless, some changes are relatively easy to forecast: these are reviewed in the first section of this chapter. Technical possibilities cannot, however, be divorced from the policy context within which they must be realised. Thus if the arguments for greater concentration as put forward, for example, by NAHAT (1993) and supported by some of the evidence presented in Chapter 5 are correct, the question remains whether such a pattern can be achieved. The second section, therefore, sets out a number of scenarios for the development of acute hospital services which combine different political and technical assumptions.

On any scenario, change is inevitable: the following section, therefore, goes on to consider the obstacles to change, particularly those which inhibit the search for new ways of working and hence the range of possible 'solutions' available to managers and purchasers. The next section identifies the implications of the argument and evidence of the report as a whole for the main 'actors' – government, purchasers, providers and professions. The chapter ends with a very brief conclusion for the report as a whole.

11.1   Immediate prospects

Despite the large areas of uncertainty, some directions of change seem clear. Data presented in Chapter 9 described how hospital activity has responded to new medical technology and to economic and other pressures: these trends, if projected forward for another ten years, in themselves imply a continuing need for change in the work and organisation of acute hospitals. The most obvious trend is that towards ever shorter lengths of stay and consequent reduction in the volume of inpatient work. The decline in length of stay during the 1980s and indeed earlier was brought about by reductions across all age groups and in all specialties and diagnosis groups. There were many forces at work – improvements in management such as better bed utilisation, medical technology, particularly anaesthesia, diagnostic techniques, new forms of treatment and within the latter, day care, particularly in surgery, itself made possible by medical advances and better organisation. All these will continue to work at shortening the average length of stay.

Although the growth of day care has been rapid, there is a long way to go, even if no further developments in medical technology take place. During the 1980s, the switch to day care was much slower than was clinically and organisationally possible (Merry, 1990). The Audit Commission's report on day surgery (1991) revealed a range of obstacles that had prevented more rapid implementation, most of which could be removed by better management.

There are now many signs that a determined attempt is being made to remove these obstacles. The NHS Executive Task Force was established to promote it, and many purchasers are requiring specified proportions of total activity to be performed on a day basis. *The Guidance to Purchasers* (Department of Health 1994) has emphasised the desirability of setting such targets. Although it remains hard to make precise forecasts, these measures, combined with the prospects of further technological advance discussed in Chapter 9, seem set to ensure that three-quarters or more of surgery will be done on a day basis and lengths of stay for the remaining work will also fall.

Within the medical specialties, length of stay also fell during the 1980s, but it is less easy to forecast confidently that it will continue to come down. The main reason for being cautious is the continuing rise in emergency admissions, which in some areas has led to rising lengths of stay and the re-introduction of bed capacity. Nevertheless, further declines may be expected, as less efficient providers catch up with the more efficient and as conscious bed management and discharge policies are more generally adopted, and also as the scope for developing community-based alternatives is further explored.

In her review of discharge procedures, Marks (1993) pointed to persistent failures in hospital discharge planning and also a large number of ways in which the process can be improved;, most lie in the field of management and organisation – though some, such as the financial framework for long term care do not. The Audit Commission (1993) reached a similar conclusion. On this basis, there would seem to be a large amount of scope for further reductions in the length of hospital stays and that, set against the modest rate of growth in the number of hospital episodes implied by any feasible projection of the funds likely to be available to the NHS, implies a further reduction in the need for beds and a further reduction in the acute hospital's role as an inpatient facility.

Important though these changes are, they do not undermine the role of the acute general hospital. Indeed, as they reflect increases in efficiency, they tend to strengthen it. Thus if the existing trends continued, the result would be more work – measured in terms of episodes – using new techniques such as minimal access surgery, and absorbing fewer (non-medical) resources per episode of care. Some work would move to other settings through accelerated discharge, relocation of outpatient services (but these would still employ hospital-based staff) and further contracting-out for services such as pathology. Changes such as these would serve to emphasise the role of the acute general hospital as a quick turnover provider of episodic care, consultation and diagnosis.

Furthermore, acute general hospitals retain considerable strengths which may well allow their business to expand: they will remain the sole providers of a number of health technologies and procedures, particularly intensive care. They may be the site of specialist units focusing on particular groups of patient such as stroke victims, even if much of their work takes place outside the boundaries of the hospital itself.

There remains an excess demand for some of their services and little sign that resources will increase fast enough to remove it; they can protect their market by themselves developing some of the alternative forms of service considered here; developments in medical technology are as likely to create further demand for hospital services as the reverse. They have shown themselves able to reduce costs and improve quality of service and there is scope for further improvement in both, through greater operational efficiency, through developments of new ways of deploying staff and possibly also through greater professional specialisation.

At the same time, the acute general hospital is threatened from a number of sources:

- intermediate units carrying out a wide range of functions now carried out in district general hospitals, particularly diagnosis, simple surgery and some inpatient medical care;
- GP surgeries and local health centres also taking on some of these functions;
- home-based care – including self medication and hospital-at-home – leading to loss of some work altogether or reduced use of inpatient facilities;
- private suppliers of ancillary services developing in areas such as pathology or recuperation facilities;

- mobile resources, eg home visitors, district nurses and practice nurses, enlarging their role and reducing the need for referrals.

The analysis set out in Chapter 4 suggested that over a considerable range of functions, hospitals and other providers will be competing to provide services that are separable from core acute facilities or substitutable by other modes But the evidence to show which mode is best in this competitive area is not generally available. As a consequence, the boundaries between hospitals and other institutions will be fuzzy, subject to change in both directions and may well vary as between different parts of the country.

Some developments could threaten, and indeed are already threatening, the viability of particular units over the full range of general hospital functions. A report from the NHS Anglia and Oxford Region (1995) floated the idea of a general hospital without accident and emergency facilities. In other parts of the country, attempts are being made to define viable local hospitals which fall short of the full range of DGH services but which have a larger role than the community hospital range described in Chapter 1. In London and other cities, the forces described in Chapter 9, particularly those relating to the medical labour market, are leading to proposals for reductions in the number of sites from which emergency care is offered and also for consolidation of smaller specialist units into large ones.

Such consolidation is largely supported by professional judgement operating within the constraints of current medical staffing policies, current technologies, and financial pressures. The evidence presented in Chapter 5 provides some degree of support for such changes. But that evidence does not show how far on purely clinical grounds such consolidation should be taken nor what the costs of access or provision resulting from it may be.

The fact that no 'solution' to these issues has emerged from this report cannot be ascribed solely to poor evidence. It also arises because the availability of options is increasing, partly as a result of new technology, partly because major restrictions on how hospitals work, particularly the division of work between professionals and the requirements of medical training, may become less binding. Consequently, new forms of service delivery relying, for example, on developments in IT and data transfer and new professional roles may emerge which will allow combination, of quality, access and cost, which are not currently feasible. Furthermore, although the factors discussed in Chapter 9 are impelling change, the changes that can emerge are also dependent on a wider range of factors than those considered so far and it is these we consider next.

11.2 The context for change

When the 1962 Plan was drawn up, it was possible for a Minister to consider setting a blueprint for the whole country – subject to the availability of resources. Even so, central direction from the Department of Health was not consistently applied: in large measure, Regions went their own way drawing up their own strategies, choosing their own regional specialties and their own hospital designs. They were able to influence the direction and location of developments through their control over capital funds. No hospital, or its managing health authority, had direct access to capital funds: cases had to be put 'through Region'. Accordingly, the regional level planners were able to exercise substantial influence. Within that framework, considerable change took place both in the workload of the hospital and the way it was executed and managed.

In the 1990s, the context within which hospital planners work is different: the forces making for change look, if anything, stronger than ever, while the context within which those forces will realise themselves looks to be more flexible and responsive, in large measure due to the NHS and Community Care Act 1990.

This did not bear directly on the role of hospitals: the preceding white paper *Working for Patients* was concerned with structures for delivering care rather than the care itself. As a consequence, the creation of both purchasing authorities and trusts has taken place with little or no depth of analysis of the issues discussed in this report. Nevertheless, introduction of the new regime did open the way for change in the role of hospitals by altering the framework within which they work, and hence the incentives of the various actors within the health care sector as a whole. The principal changes are these:

- there is greater potential for competition between hospitals under the new arrangements than existed before 1990 as a result of the introduction of the purchaser/provider split;
- the way is more open than it has been hitherto for a switch in resources between hospitals and other uses or indeed vice versa;
- there is more scope for changes to take place in the mode of delivery of what are now hospital services since trusts have greater freedom to determine reward and staffing structures;
- the introduction of capital charges has created an incentive to reduce reliance on capital - intensive modes of provision and hence to reduce physical capacity wherever possible;
- the introduction of fundholding has created effective pressure on hospitals to change the way in which they delivery services;

- centrally imposed efficiency targets and the requirements of the *Patient's Charter*, particularly on waiting times, have created further pressures to improve performance.

As a result, the policy environment within which hospitals now work is a much more demanding one than it was prior to 1991. Combined with the economic and technological pressures described earlier, they underline the inevitability of change. But although the context within which hospitals operate is more flexible than it was prior to 1990, there are obstacles to change which could limit the scope for hospitals and other providers to respond to the new opportunities apparently open to them..

Financial structures

While in principle district purchasers are in a position to shift finance for hospital services to wherever they consider they are best applied, that does not apply to family health services. As things stand, there is no financial incentive for GPs to take on more work from hospitals nor means of paying them if they do beyond the modest payments made for running disease-specific clinics. Equally, payments from the general medical services budget are tied to general practitioners so that other potential providers of general medical services cannot enter the market except in very limited circumstances, eg special schemes to serve the homeless. Such schemes as exist typically draw on special or experimental budgets, not mainstream funding.

Weaknesses in primary care

General practitioners are now able to offer a wider range of services within their own premises and envisage taking on even more. In some parts of the country that does not hold: practices are small and poorly equipped. In London, for example, a primary care development zone has been set up in an attempt to improve practice standards – ie to make sure, in the current phrase, that the basics are right before attention is paid to the more ambitious task of absorbing work now done in hospitals.

Market structure

While the introduction of the purchaser/provider split and the subsequent market behaviour it has given rise to are two of the main factors likely to lead to change, there are significant tensions between market processes and the achievement of a particular pattern of hospital services. These arise on both the demand and the supply side of the market.

On the demand side, a central difficulty was identified by the Clinical Standards Advisory Group. The Group's report (1993) on specialist services expressed their concern that the funding of such units might become insecure under the new arrangements since they rely on attracting custom from a large number of purchasers. In fact, they found no evidence of any adverse effects so far but the same risks arise with any function, including research and training, which relies on attracting custom from a large number of purchasers, some of whom are making only occasional demands on the service.

Despite the risks identified in this report, the Department of Health continues to reduce the scale of 'high-level' purchasing. As noted in Chapter 1, until recently the Department of Health funded directly a number of national centres of specialised care and Regional Health Authorities other centres. Now the policy (NHSME 1993) is to actively promote the break-up of that system in favour of 'lead' purchasers and multi-purchaser arrangements.

Thus, one way or other, if the clinical and cost arguments for greater concentration of some services are accepted, then some meta-level purchaser is required or some effective means has to be found for co-ordinating purchasing plans. Such co-ordination can be achieved by agreement and may not need to be 'enforced' but it may not prove feasible, depending as it would on goodwill.

However, the effect of going down this route would be to produce a pattern of hospital services which was highly monopolistic and within which the scope for market behaviour was very limited. Only on the fringes of catchment areas would competition be effective. In such an environment, either new forms of competition would have to be introduced (Propper 1995) or other strategies introduced to maintain the pressure for improved quality and lower costs.

There is the further implication that the present structure of trusts is not appropriate to the pattern of services that some of the evidence presented here, particularly in Chapter 6, suggests might be most effective. Boyle and Harrison (1995) have argued that this could mean that the future of the acute hospital might have to be thought of in terms of services rather than institutions and if that is right, the present structure of provision represents an obstacle to change, since it encourages competition where co-operation may be more appropriate.

Human resources

Changes of the kind this report suggests are likely in the pattern of hospital provision will require large changes in skills, professional roles and the boundaries between professions.

Similarly, the development of new community-based services and a closer fusion between primary and secondary care will only take root if there are health service professionals who are actively interested in developing new forms of provision and who are prepared to challenge and rethink established ways of working. While many are, others, it would appear, are not.

Within hospitals themselves, changes in medical staffing structures are inevitable, as the Government has now explicitly recognised in respect of junior doctors. But there remain significant barriers to changes in the way medical and other professional staff are used within hospitals. Perhaps the most important, as already suggested in Chapter 9, are the constraints imposed by the requirements of medical training. Others, as the Audit Commission (1995) has pointed out, stem from tradition and custom. The examples cited in Chapter 9 indicate that the barriers posed by tradition are beginning to crumble.

Public opinion:

The trends and possibilities set out above imply a future in which change is continuous and existing institutions are threatened. The public in general are highly attached to 'their' hospital: reductions in beds or worse, closures, are automatically opposed. As a report from NHS South Thames (1994) indicates, it is now virtually impossible to close a district general hospital. Although the Secretary of State has approved closures in London, in other areas closures or major reconfigurations have been dropped in the face of a hostile public.

The central technical difficulty is that at present the arguments which would justify a change in the pattern of acute care are poorly understood – in the terms used by Virginia Bottomley when Secretary of State for Health in another context – the public is not 'health literate'. There is little general awareness of the weaknesses in the existing pattern of provision and hence as a consequence, change is going to continue to be resisted, however good the arguments for it. Some of the measures suggested in the following section, particularly the release of more information about hospital services, will help. But the issue goes much deeper than that: the hospital embodies in its physical presence, however dilapidated or brutish its exterior appearance, and however great the risks it actually imposes on its users, a source of safety when a threat to life occurs. It is a source of reassurance, particularly potent in the present political climate in which neither the Government nor individual purchasers are trusted to maintain services. Hospital closure is one of the few local issues which will pack public meetings and bring people on to the streets. 'Closer to home' has its own reassuring ring, but it lacks the physical image that the hospital inherently possesses.

11.3   Some scenarios for hospital development

The analytic framework set out in Chapters 2 and 3 implicitly assumed that some organisation would be in a position to 'play God' and impose whatever was seen to be the 'best' pattern of hospital provision. In practice, of course, change has to be effected within a given institutional framework and that, as the previous section showed, is not one in which central planning for the hospital system as a whole has a role.

The rest of this section aims to bring out some of the relationships between the policy framework and the system – primarily the hospital system – it is intended to influence through a series of scenarios which pair up alternative views of the future pattern of health care delivery with alternative policy frameworks.

1: Continue as now

The immediate prospect is for a continuing rationalisation of acute capacity, leading to disposals of land and buildings, and pressures to provide finance to maintain existing institutions or face the costs – financial and political – of major restructuring This should produce steady if unspectacular improvements in performance, but possibly at a faster rate. It would allow some locational and some mode substitution of existing hospital services. The major question marks over *Continue as now* arise in two main areas:

- whether the existing purchasing structure can achieve radical change. In some cases, purchasers should be able to reap benefits of scale, particularly in the case of elective surgery, if they are provided to override the interests of their local providers. But purchasers as at present constituted will find it hard to implement the kind of structural changes that, for example, the Government's proposals for cancer services involve.
- whether existing providers, either community trusts or general practitioners, will be able to develop services which substitute for those now provided within hospitals. Many are experimenting with such services but such experiments remain small scale, in part because of financial obstacles to more fundamental change, in part because purchasers continue to protect 'their' acute hospital.

2: Planned structural change

Such an approach seems the very antithesis of the present policy framework and hence unlikely short of a change of government. However, as experience in London has shown, the present Government has felt it necessary to intervene to preserve certain institutions and, if the pressures, either political or clinical, were great enough would no doubt do so more generally. It is the appropriate approach if large-scale reconfiguration is desired.

The main weaknesses of this scenario are:

- the knowledge base is not yet strong enough to support it. As the present authors argued in *Health Care UK 1993/94*, a national blueprint, an updated version of the 1962 Plan, is not appropriate since the fundamental trade-offs vary from area to area. Furthermore, the currently available information is not sufficiently strong to define a blueprint which could be applied as a national policy.
- the organisational and planning capacity to implement a central view does not exist. The Government is intent on reducing the numbers of staff at HQ and regional level and, as a consequence, much of the capacity that once existed will soon disappear.

However, relevant evidence will accumulate and some of the measures that the Government has itself taken, such as those in relation to junior hospital medical staff, will compel change. It may become clear that it is ineffective and costly to retain general hospitals in some parts of the country and that benefits are to be won by creating new structures of provision, in physical and organisational terms. Thus in time, this option may begin to impose itself as indeed it has to some degree in London.

3: Rapid development of market processes

The central difficulty here is to imagine what is actually meant by a market in the UK health care sector, given the existing constraints on finance imposed on public sector bodies like trusts. Under present policies, the most likely development of market forces would come about from further development of the private finance initiative and some degree of competitive tendering for clinical services.

On this basis, the most likely source of new facilities is a joint public/private venture. So far, the effect of the private finance initiative has been limited to specialist services such as clinical waste disposal, apparently because the rules governing the use of private finance within the NHS, although relaxed, are still too restrictive. If they were relaxed further, the next step might be the major elective facility, perhaps based on a trust which risks losing a large amount of work to another nearby hospital. In other words, incremental, generally small-scale, projects might prove feasible.

However, over a period of time such projects could lead to substantial change in the structure of acute care. Elective work would be carried out in separate institutions or within existing ones, on a contract basis. This would lead in the direction envisaged by Boyle and Harrison (1995) of the acute hospital being a piece of infrastructure into which a range of services slot.

The major weaknesses of this scenario are:

- it is hard to see how it can achieve fundamental structural change where this involves planning services across several hospitals;
- it is hard to see how it would promote interconnections between providers of the kind that 'seamlessness' implies: indeed it would tend to make it harder to achieve by introducing further boundaries between services;
- it is hard to see how it can be maintained indefinitely if it is correct that some services will enjoy natural monopolies.

4: Halfway house – major intervention to achieve some specific objectives

The Government's acceptance of the case for a network of cancer services implies recognition of the need for limited intervention to achieve national policy goals. In fact, the expert report and the government circular issued with it did not specify an implementation mechanism, but if purchasers fail to agree locally on what the pattern of care should be, then pressure could well develop for central intervention. The main weaknesses of this scenario are implicit in those already discussed;

- the knowledge is not strong enough to support it;
- the capacity to implement it is not in place.

The main point the scenarios serve to identify is that there are tensions, unrecognised when the NHS and Community Care Act (1990) was drafted, between the appropriate structure of supply of hospitals services, and the market processes the 1990 reforms were designed to develop. If core acute services continue to concentrate on fewer sites, and particularly if these are linked contractually through arrangements such as hub and spoke, then the implicit assumptions underlying the reforms will cease to hold. The Government can, as in the public utilities, go down the regulatory road: the first signs of a move in this direction are to be found in *Managing the Internal Market* (Department of Health, 1994). Or it can rethink the nature and role of trusts in relation to hospital provision and with that the nature of the medical labour market and possibly that for other professions as well.

To another government, less interested in competition, the scenarios offer a different direction, towards a greater or less degree of intervention to achieve particular service structures. But here again the existing structure of NHS organisation present obstacles to implementing it.

11.4   Action required

In the course of this report, a number of areas have been identified where some form of initiative or change is required. This concluding section groups them according to the agency responsible for taking action.

Department of Health/NHS

Finance: The way that finance is provided does not facilitate purchasers to search for the best pattern of care nor does it recognise the strains that major shifts in the pattern of care delivery will impose. The fixed point of the current system – the self-employed GP, with funding tied to the 1990 contract – is a central obstacle to the development of new forms of provision outside hospitals. Currently GPs' remuneration is largely tied to the General Medical Services Contract. They can be paid more by other purchasers in respect of work outside that role, eg if they act as clinical assistants within hospitals, but not if extra work arising from changes within the acute hospital's role extends 'normal' GP work. If boundaries between providers are to be flexible, a way must be found of removing this obstacle.

Access: Radical change in the structure of hospital provision will pose access difficulties for some sections of the population. While a lot can be done to change the location of some hospital services so as to improve access, greater concentration of others will worsen it. The policy issue here is whether the existing rules governing provision of transport to hospitals and of financial support towards the costs of travel will be adequate and, if quality demands greater concentration of hospital work than now obtains, that will be recognised in the formula governing the allocation of finance to purchasers. As pointed out in Chapter 9, different policies currently operate in different parts of the UK and in different services. GPs' payments comprise a sparsity weighting but hospital and community services do not, at least within England, though they receive one in other parts of the UK. Shifts in care away from the acute hospital would undermine this distinction. Equally, if the pressures for concentration could only be resisted in rural areas by supporting high cost units, then there would be a case for recognising this in the national allocation formula.

Purchasing Structure: There is currently no clear policy of what the structure of purchasing should be. On the one hand, the Government is supporting smaller purchasers, such as GP fundholders, while permitting the creation of commissions covering larger areas on the other. As argued already, neither has been designed against an explicit view as to how the hospital sector is going to develop. If the ' hierarchical system' approach is valid, be it for accident and emergency, cancer or any other service, then the Government must be confident that purchasing structures are adequate to realise it. At present it cannot be.

Outcome Measures: The NHS Executive has now introduced performance measures for hospitals but they do not bear on the central issues discussed here. For good reasons the Executive has been reluctant to publish crude death rates – though they have been published in Scotland: unadjusted they are misleading and the appropriate adjustments are hard to make. Nevertheless, the measurement of clinical quality must be addressed. What that needs is a much more systematic analysis of current hospital activity.

At present even the existing sources are not fully exploited. Chapters 5 and 9 drew on existing data to shed some light on how the present system of hospital provision works. The data are subject to a number of weaknesses and limitations, some of which could be easily corrected, others would take substantial extra time and resources. But there is no reason why in the interim it should not be systematically used to monitor how the use of the hospital system is changing. Furthermore, existing sources could be the basis of a systematic monitoring of outcomes, based, perhaps, on samples of cases in particularly critical areas. In other words, a new system of centralised audit is required if outcomes are to be taken seriously.

Research: A large number of areas where further research is needed have been identified, some of which is under way.The Executive is supporting a programme of research on the interface between primary and secondary care, which should illuminate many of the issues identified here, particularly in the area of substitution and the role of intermediate institutions. But this does not bear on the central role of the hospital and the conditions under which hospital care is best provided.

These are very difficult areas to research because so many factors need to be taken into account simultaneously. But while the majority of the nation's resources continue to be used in hospitals, their effectiveness as providers of care should be addressed. Many individual topics are being tackled, such as day surgery, but the central structural issues remain strangely neglected in the Department of Health's research programme. As argued elsewhere (Harrison, 1996), this omission reflects a general bias in favour of 'micro' research, involving detailed examination of narrowly defined issues. As a result, issues which cut across the boundaries of traditional subjects or which require the scope of the research to be very wide – as with hospital structures – are neglected.

There is no agreed way of comparing the merits of alternative configurations of specialties. In principle, the merits of particular clusters should be measurable, or at minimum it should be possible to identify the number and types of patients which might benefit or lose out from different clusters. But no such information is either routinely available nor regularly presented when changes in acute care are proposed.

Competition Policy: Closely linked to the issue of purchasing structure is the question of whether or not competition should be preserved in the face of the monopolistic implications of the creation of units serving large areas. As our scenarios have emphasised, three options exist:

- to keep concentration below the maximum which medical and other arguments might justify trading quality off against cost, over time;
- to promote concentration and consider other means of promoting competition, eg through tendering for the right to provide or manage services: that would require a revolution in the way that medical staff was employed, turning it, in effect, into a hired resource, like catering;
- to live with lack of competition and go down the regulatory route adopted for public utilities. That would involve privatising supply and use of direct or indirect profit control to avoid exploitation.

Managing the New NHS (Department of Health 1993c) ducked these substantive issues in favour of a (largely desirable) organisational streamlining. *The Operation of the NHS Internal Market* (NHS Management Executive, 1994) began the process of defining a regulatory regime, but left a large number of issues unanswered, particularly those surrounding the maintenance of competitive pressures and the issue of new entry.

A change of government may lead to a change of policy, including perhaps rejection of markets and competition. But the central issue which the 1990 Act attempted to address – how to get more of a limited volume of health resources – will not go away, so the need for some form of pressure, to use an alternative word, for better performance will persist. This may require some institutional innovation on the lines suggested by Boyle and Harrison (1995) which would involve introducing competition below the level of the individual trust hospital, but other means are possible. In the education sector, for example, poorly performing schools can be 'taken over', but such extreme sanctions have not yet been seriously considered for health services.

Implications for purchasers

The central implication for purchasers is clear and familiar: look for evidence of outcomes. The evidence presented above, subject to certain statistical health warnings, suggests that better outcomes will tend to be associated with higher volumes in some areas of hospital work. It also suggests that certain configurations and staffing arrangements tend to promote better outcomes or at least make them easier or cheaper to achieve.

This evidence, much of it from other hospital systems, is only a starting point, for the reasons set out in Chapter 5. But while it may not be strong enough to compel wholesale transfers of care, it does serve to emphasise the need to define the conditions where the chances of getting the best possible level of care are highest and to identify areas of current poor performance. At present, it is hard for purchasers to follow this advice, and indeed few are staffed appropriately to do so.

Our analysis also points up the importance of access: if concentration is promoted, then the issue of access must be addressed and become an explicit and central part of purchasing policy. Many purchasers are expressing concern over access but there is little routine information published or analysed on what access patterns are. That may mean *ad hoc* data collection or better use of existing sources (Benzeval, 1995). Admission data can be used to map the utilisation of particular facilities and in conjunction with travel time and public transport information, *prima facie* evidence of travel difficulties can be assembled. But much more detailed work is required drawing on population-based epidemiological information to show whether it is physical access or other obstacles which are affecting utilisation rates (Majeed, 1994).

Implications for hospital providers

The overall message of this report is not a comfortable one for providers of acute hospital services since it threatens existing levels of demand, emphasises the need for continuing change even if current levels of demand persist and the overall uncertainty within which they will inevitably operate. There are threats for both large and small acute hospitals.

For the smaller institutions, the threats suggested by the evidence in favour of greater scale and higher thresholds for emergency care are clear. But new forms of staffing and new technology, particularly in communications and information, can help to counter them. For the larger institutions, particularly those which dominate their local market, the threats they face may seem literally marginal. But they will not be immune from many of the pressures for change identified in this report: for lower costs, better measures of outcomes and changes in the way that services are provided.

Implications for other providers

The opportunity to capture what is now hospital business is clear in the areas defined in Chapters 3 and 4 as separable from core acute facilities and/or substitutable by other providers. However, with very few exceptions, the benefits of changes in provider have yet to be rigorously demonstrated in ways which combine clinical considerations with those of cost and access. The way forward, therefore, is for incremental change accompanied by clinical and consumer audit.

The professions

This report has drawn extensively on documents produced by groups of professionals, typically within one medical specialty. Each recognise the central challenge – to demonstrate which configuration of services gives the greatest chance of good quality care.

Typically, however, they suffer from four weaknesses:

- they take a service or specialty at a time, each representing an ideal view for that specialty, without explicit reference to the resource implications of their general adoption or to the implications for the hospital as a whole. Thus they allow no scope for effective dialogue across the spectrum of medical specialties, still less all the professionals involved. But it is precisely the links between specialties and different professionals which make or break the case for different configurations of acute services;

- many of the basic judgements made are implicit, so that the trade-offs being made are unclear. Access standards are usually proposed with no supporting evidence either on their rationale or the implied costs of imposing them. Equally, the value put on risk avoidance which is implicit in standards set for staffing levels and the availability of equipment is typically unspecified;
- information on costs is rarely offered;
- typically, proposals are based on professional judgements rather than research or audit results.

As a result, the professions manage to avoid what the analysis of Chapters 3 and 4 suggested are the central issues for hospital planning – the links between the different activities which acute care requires.

Medical training

The hospital has been, and still frequently is, primarily regarded as an organisation designed for the education and training of medical staff. That clearly has to change. The relationship between hospital and the training of medical staff has to alter whatever the precise pattern of hospital provision. At present hospitals in general, but smaller hospitals in particular, are held back from developing new forms of staffing lest some of their posts lose recognition for training purposes from the Royal Colleges. The Colleges are in this respect strictly non-responsible. There is no line of accountability for the reasonableness of these requirements and so no forum within which their cost, in the broadest sense, can be assessed.

Medical education itself will have to change. Medical schools are already moving towards the concept of the 'teaching district' rather than the 'teaching hospital'. Within that broader concept, all health care providers, whatever their institutional attachment, have a part to play, as *Widening the Horizons of Medical Education* (King's Fund 1994) suggested.

> *There are major pressure towards a community defined curriculum which will be responsive to the needs of the local population rather than the perceived needs of the [medical] school itself. (p 1)*

Extra-hospital and inter-professional linkages are growing in importance relative to intra-hospital and intra-professional linkages. Teaching will have to follow, not determine, the pattern of provision. The Medical Workforce Standing Advisory Committee has expressed the view, cited in Chapter 9, that some providers may wish to opt out of the training role. In that way, they may be freer to adopt innovative staffing structures and working methods.

11.5 Overall conclusion

Acute hospital providers are facing a time of extreme turbulence. It is not clear in exactly what their future role will be, but they will not be allowed the luxury of standing still to find out. In the course of this report, a number of different ways of defining their role have emerged: a means of encouraging beneficial interaction between clinicians; a device for assembling patients for teaching purposes; a device for reducing risk and for simplifying decision-making for others; and a managed infrastructure into which services organised by others can plug. The fundamental question for the future of the general hospital is: which of these roles will continue to be vital for the well-functioning of the health care system as a whole?

As Rosemary Stevens (1989) puts it in *In Sickness and in Wealth*, her study of the American hospital:

> . . . the hospital is not an inevitable institution. It is forged by individuals and it is sensitive to economic incentives and to other cultural rewards and disincentives – the messages, that is, in its immediate environment. There is no set design for the hospital's organisational role or for the structure or performance of the hospital system. (p14)

Whatever the overall merits of the 1990 reforms, they have at least opened up directions that were, in the 'old' NHS, unthinkable – new possible trajectories, in Stevens' words. The process of re-inventing the hospital may as a result be promoted rather than held back. It remains, nonetheless, perhaps a greater challenge than the reforms themselves.

Annex

Terminology and Data Sources

Most official documents do not attempt definitions of either hospital or acute care nor of primary/secondary/community. Acute care is commonly defined as care provided when the condition of the patient requires an immediate, or at least an urgent response, ie within a few days. But what are called acute hospitals in fact provide care for conditions for which are not serious and often do so to a leisurely timescale. And, outside the hospital itself, care may be provided by health care professionals or paramedics to deal with serious life threatening conditions.

Sometimes definitions are offered in terms of level of skill or technology. The hospital is the place for high-tech medicine and the highest levels of human skills. But again, examples can be found where both are matched outside the hospital itself. Some have seen the essence of the hospital as the intensive care facility, but many hospitals do not possess one. Some see the hospital as a place where complex (medical) work gets done but some hospitals concentrate on work that would not normally be called complex.

Paralleling the acute/non-acute division is that between primary and secondary. In the UK and other health systems with a highly developed system of general practice, to which people normally turn in the first instance, the notions of primary as 'first contact' and 'routine' or 'basic' care have merged. But some hospital services, particularly accident and emergency may be termed primary care since they represent the first point of contact for the patient and are provided on an open-access basis while some GP work is neither 'routine' nor 'basic'. In what follows, however, we will use primary care only for services provided by general practitioners and their staff, including nurses and other professionals under their direction.

- Services managed by the hospital but provided outside it is termed hospital outreach.
- Care provided in the home is termed hospital at home or domiciliary care.
- Facilities such as polyclinics, community hospitals etc are termed intermediate facilities.

Although these definitions – or better, perhaps, working conventions – are some assistance, they fall short of defining what a hospital actually is. Most of this report is about the institutions which call themselves (acute general) hospitals and which provide acute care in response to demands for immediate treatment but which will also provide a range of service, from elective inpatient treatment, rehabilitation and diagnostics, which are not themselves meeting acute needs. What these are in the UK can be discovered by looking at the index of the *Health Services Yearbook*. But for analytic purposes this ostensive definition will not do. Once alternative dispositions of activities which currently take place in these institutions are considered, a decision has to be made whether the nomenclature 'hospital' follows the activities, as in 'hospital at home' or whether the essence of the hospital resides in the institution.

For analytic purposes, the hospital in this report is treated as a large cluster of health care facilities, a definition which means that a group practice would count as a (small) hospital. Confusing though that would be in everyday speech, for present purposes that implication is acceptable, since the central and recurring question throughout the report is what activities should be clustered together. That question is as relevant to the group practice as it is to 'the hospital'.

Finally, it is just as hard to define *a* hospital. Within the NHS, in some parts of the country, hospitals are managed in groups. Before the reforms that was done by a single district, after them by a single trust. This means care has to be taken to distinguish physical proximity such as a single site creates from organisational proximity which a single management may, or may not, provide.

In some cases, physical proximity is critical and hence the narrow definition of a hospital confining it to one site is significant. In others, it is not, and the precise physical extent of *a* hospital, is immaterial: what matters is the organisational framework linking services on different sites. Unfortunately, the way in which UK hospitals are described for statistical purposes has veered from one definition to another in recent years: until recently a very small amount of data was available for individual sites: most applied to the managing district health authority. With the creation of trusts, most nationally collected data refer to provider units, some of which operate on single sites; others do not. Some providers operate only acute care facilities, others also provide long stay and community facilities of various kinds. In practice then, the distinction between site and management unit is virtually impossible to make.

The reader would be right to conclude that it would be sensible to abandon the word hospital and talk only in terms of services and sites for service delivery. That may, at some stage, be a sensible approach but at the present time it seems wiser to continue with the terms in present use.

The difficulties in definition are compounded by deficiencies in respect of data. Anyone attempting a statistical description of the hospital system in the UK is immediately thwarted by the lack of consistent definitions and published series. Anyone attempting to do the same for the largest part of it, ie England, runs into similar difficulties of which the most important was the change made in the mid-1980s to the way that hospital-based statistics were compiled. The measure of activity commonly used changed from the district stay to the finished consultant episode. That meant an immediate apparent increase in activity, since many hospital stays consist of several episodes, as the Department of Health Statistical Bulletin, *Acute Hospital Activity*, reveal. These *Bulletins* are nevertheless useful for the recent past; for further back, Department of Health and Social Security (1981) and Tew (1976) are helpful, but neither deals with individual hospitals or procedures.

In this report we have focused primarily upon England, but drawn, from time to time on data from Scotland since the Scots did not follow England in changing the basis of hospital statistics in the mid-1980s and also because they publish a great deal more information about their hospitals. There are significant differences between Scotland and England, not least the higher level of per capita spend in the smaller country, but as far as the nature of the hospital services and the changes occurring within them, it seems a reasonable assumption that Scotland and England are broadly similar.

Despite their central position, there is no adequate description, as far as England in particular is concerned, of the work hospitals do which bears on the structure of provision as opposed to the overall level of activity. The Department of Health does not publish data on the workload of individual hospitals or provider units in England, nor does it, or its counterparts in the other three countries, publish information on individual categories of work, ie particular treatments or procedures, showing in what setting it is done. Thus there is no way of showing from published sources whether or not there is a sharp dividing line between the work done in general hospitals and that done elsewhere,nor between the district general hospital and the larger referral centres.

Chapter 5 draws on unpublished information derived from individual patient records. Most records contain a procedure or diagnostic code. The number of diagnoses and procedures in current use in the UK is far too large for present purposes. Instead, we draw on analysis by health-resource groups have been used, of which some 500 or so are currently in use. These group together diagnoses and procedures with similar clinical and resource use characteristics. The analysis includes all provider units carrying out some elements of acute care and has been made available to us on an anonymised basis, ie individual hospitals cannot be identified. The data used by the National Case-Mix Office combine trusts and what were in 1992/3 directly managed units. Both may comprise what were earlier counted as more than one district hospital.

Bibliographical notes

All the sources cited in the text are listed below. However, the bibliography also contains a number of sources not explicitly cited in the text but which have been found helpful either as background or as providing evidence confirming that in the sources which have been cited. In what follows, we draw attention to some of these references and also to sources which provide a more detailed coverage of some of the issues covered in this report.

The literature on the acute hospital is best described as fragmented. With a very few exceptions, the recent literature , except that concerned with hospital management, focuses on part of the work of the hospital rather than the hospital as a whole. The bulk of the literature which does consider the hospital as a whole and its place in the health care sector is short on evidence and the areas covered by systematic reviews of the literature remain few.

Chapter I

The development of hospitals and hospital policy over the last 30 years is poorly served in the literature. The period prior to the NHS is covered in Abel-Smith (1964), the inter-war period by Gray (1991) and the period from 1948 to 1960 by Webster (1988). The period since the formulation of the 1962 Plan is not comprehensively covered in any one source, but useful material can be found in Allen (1976 and 1979), Klein (1989) and Ham (1982). There is no comprehensive source on the district general hospital. Dowie's series of studies (1989–1991) is not easy reading, but it provides a unique insight into the way that medical staffing in general hospitals of various kinds actually works. So also does the report on gastroenterology services in Gut (1989).

As Fox (1986) brings out, in some ways the US and the UK have developed under similar influences even if in others they are very different. Stevens (1989) provides a description on the development of the American hospital in the 20th century which discusses some of the factors, such as growth of medical knowledge, which affect both systems. No British source comes close to Stevens but Granshaw (1992) tells part of the story.

As far as 'small' or community hospitals are concerned, both Tucker (1987) and Higgins (1993) provide useful overviews and, in the latter case, an extensive bibliography. The Royal College of Surgeons (1985) gives a succinct résumé of the factors explaining the decline of the community hospital during the 1980s. Some further references not cited in the text are: Ramaiah (1994) and Jones *et al* 1988).

As this report was being prepared for the press, a wide-ranging survey of the role of the hospital (Vetter 1995) was published. Although the subject is ostensibly the same as that of this report, the treatment is so different that their coverage rarely overlaps. This source is particularly useful as a source of examples of some of the general points made here, particularly as it draws on a wider range of clinical material.

Chapter 2

The arguments discussed in this chapter can be found in the official reports listed in Table 1.1 and some of them received a more thorough airing in the 1960s and 1970s, particularly in the Bonham-Carter report (Department of Health and Social Security/Welsh Office 1969) than they have done subsequently in official publications. As far as recent texts are concerned, Dixon *et al* (1992) and South East Thames Regional Health Authority (1991) are the best introductions to thinking about the hospital as a whole, but the more recent report from the NHS Anglia and Oxford Region (1995b), though focused on emergency services, also raises issues about the structure of the hospital as a whole.

In general, the specialty or service rather than the hospital has been the main 'unit of analysis'. This chapter and the following one therefore draws on a number of reports from specialty groups usually within one or other of the Royal Colleges or the *ad hoc* groups which prepared reports for the London Implementation Group. These by their very nature do not address some of the issues considered in this chapter, but they normally consider questions of linkages to other specialties and to common hospital facilities. All the London Implementation Group reports are helpful in this respect as far as specialist services are concerned. The review of children's services is particularly illuminating. As this report points out, children's hospitals were typically free-standing institutions located primarily with a view to the availability of wet nurses. Although, with only a few exceptions, children's services are now to be found in general hospitals, they remain in a sense a hospital within a hospital since the view has increasingly been accepted that children should be segregated from adults in both wards and accident and emergency departments. Even where professionals also deal with adults, the report suggests their work should be overseen by those exclusively treating children. This report also draws on interesting material on the views of parents particularly those relating to the relative importance of quality and access.

The economic concepts can be found in any economics textbook, although economies of scope are less commonly discussed. Two of the seminal articles are Teece (1980) and Willig (1979): see also Bailey and Friedlander (1982).

The notion of access as part of the price of any good has been commonplace since Becker (1965) and has been extensively used in the transport field since the 1960s through the concept of generalised cost, a notion which combines money outlays on fares etc with the price of time. What the price of time should be has its own large literature: see for example MVA (1987). In the case of health, see for example Coffey (1983), McGurk and Porrell (1984), and the studies cited therein. Joseph and Phillis (1984) cover a number of areas where access costs bear on health services.

The notion of accessibility to health care goes wider than transport costs and in this wider sense it is analysed in some detail by Frenk (1985): see also Benzeval (1995).

Chapter 3

As noted above, Fox (1986) traces the notion of hierarchy in both British and American thinking about the hospital. The notion of a hierarchy can be found in all the service reviews from which this report draws, particularly the London Implementation Group reports, as these are largely concerned with those services which not all district general hospitals would be expected to have. They also cite interesting material on the relationship between different levels in the various hierarchies they set out. As noted in the text, it is sometimes proposed that the division of roles between them should be based on protocols: for a review of their effectiveness see Dukes and Stewart (1993). The implications of hierarchical arrangements for purchasing are looked at in Haward (1994).

Running through this chapter (as well as Chapter 5) is the issue of 'generalist v specialist' within hospital medical staffing. The literature on this is sparse and widely scattered and much of it lightweight. But some interesting reflections can be found in Todd (1987), Jackson (1988), Duff (1992), Barondass (1993), Greenhalg (1994), Horner *et al* (1995) and *The Lancet* (1995).

The notion that the service or specialty should be the focus of organisation of hospital (and other) services has been put forward by Malcolm in a series of articles based on experience in New Zealand where the reform of the health care sector closely mirrors the UK's 1990 reforms. A more general treatment can be found in Robinson (1994); see also Boyle and Harrison (1995).

Chapter 4

The term optimal balance used in this chapter is the title of a King's Fund report (Hughes and Gordon 1992) which describes a number of examples where the locus of care has been shifted. The concepts briefly set out in this chapter of substitution and complementarity can be found defined more rigorously in any economics textbook. In the health context, the notion of substitution is explored more widely and more systematically in Warner and Riley (1994) as well as Warner (1993). The idea that hospital use may be reduced by policies outside the hospital forms part of Fries *et al's* (1993) wider consideration of the scope for reducing expenditure on health.

The changing role of the hospital in relation to other providers is a theme common to other countries. For a transatlantic perspective, see Stoeckle (1995), Shortell *et al* (1995) and Robinson (1994).

Chapter 5

The subject of this chapter is one of the few covered in this report which has received systematic review. The sources cited in the text - Black and Johnston (1990), Flood and Scott (1987), Luft *et al* (1986), Office of Technology Assessment and NHS Centre for Reviews and Dissemination all contain extensive bibliographies as well as extensive reflections on the methodological issues involved. However they do not systematically treat the parallel literature on the benefits of specialisation within services, ie at a broader level than the individual treatment or procedure. A few examples are cited in the text; others are Stiller (1988 and 1994), Stiller and Draper (1989) and Heinemann (1989). All the London specialty reviews cited above employ arguments supporting both concentration and clustering: alternative views can be found: see for example *The Lancet* (1995), which sounds a sceptical note on the case for centralised treatment.

The area of accident and emergency services attracts an enormous literature which until recently had not been systematically reviewed. Pencheon (1995) has prepared a very extensive overview for the NHS Executive Anglia and Oxford's emergency care project and this now represents by far the best introduction currently available. The report by the Royal College of Surgeons of England (1988) also contains extensive further reading.

One of the central conclusions of this chapter is that changes in hospital configuration involve trade-offs between different groups of patient: that point, as well as other relevant to the issues discussed in this chapter, emerges from Freeland (1987). Although the quality, lost, access trichotomy can be found in many sources, attempts to apply it systematically are few: one such is McLafferty and Broe (1990).

Chapter 6

The chapter concludes with a citation from JRG Butler's (1995) study of hospital costs in Australia. This also provides a guide to many of the pitfalls of this kind of work as well as an extensive bibliography. Other sources covering a broad field are Cowing and Holtmann (1983) and Cowing *et al* (1983).

As noted in the text, clinical reviews ignore issues of cost or treat them in broad brush terms, often for lack of the relevant data. But most assume that any specialty requires a minimum size to be viable, eg the British Paediatric Association currently supports figure of 2,500 as a minimum size of a maternity unit. That suggests that costs would fall up to that point but how much beyond it is another matter.

The point is made in the text that comparisons between different types of hospital are made difficult by differences in the type of case handled. Differences in cost structure also make it difficult to interpret simple average cost differences – see for example Gray and Steel (1981) for a discussion of this point in relation to maternity care. They also make the point that differences in utilisation levels may also be important but these are to some extent a matter of policy as to where the 'slack' to cope with variability is located. Thus simple average cost comparisons, however accurate, may be beside the point.

This chapter is primarily concerned with the relationship between scale, scope and cost: for an examination of the relationship between quality and cost, see Morey *et al* (1992).

Chapter 8

The role of transport in the health sector has been overlooked in recent years. Both Rigby (1978) and Joseph and Phillips (1984) provide useful overviews even though their coverage is somewhat dated, as is Parkin and Henderson (1985). The ambulance service is poorly served by written sources; one recent overview is Sutton (1990). Pencheon's review cited above also contains relevant material as does Rousseau *et al* (1994), although its focus is on primary care. The importance of time taken to reach hospital is considered in Meyer (1979a–c), and the references cited there.

As noted above, Frenk provides a more thorough analysis of the concept of accessibility. See also Benzeval (1995) who considers different kinds of barriers to utilisation and the measures relevant to each.

Chapter 9

The changes taking place in the acute hospital briefly described here can be discerned through official sources like the Department of Health *Statistical Bulletins* on acute hospital activity and the annual statistical digest Health and Personal Social Services Statistics, but as the Annex notes, it is not always easy to match up figures from different sources nor to find a continuous series on the same basis. For many purposes, Scottish Health Statistics is more user friendly.

These difficulties to some extent explain the lack of detailed studies of hospital activity. Using the only data set which links patient records over a period of time, a number of studies have emerged for the Oxford Region for the period prior to 1986 when the basis of recording changed which describe the extent to which extra activity has extended the number of patients treated rather than the number of times the same patients are treated: see Ferguson *et al* (1991 a-c) and Goldacre *et al* (1988).

The material referred to in the text on the relationship between ageing and the use of hospital services is the tip of a very large literature. Robine *et al* (1992) contains material from a number of countries, and a trawl through recent issues of the *Milbank Quarterly* would also be useful, particularly the articles by Manton in addition to that cited in the text.

The literature of advisory referrals to hospital is large as the bibliographical material in the sources cited in the text indicate: see also Wilkin and Dorner (1990). This is not true of emergency referrals. As a result of widespread reports of increases in emergency medical admissions during 1994, a number of papers have appeared describing the changes that have taken place and attempting to pin down their causes: some examples are Kendrick (1995) and Edwards and Warneke (1994).

As noted in the main text, the scope for modal substitution of hospital care by other providers has not been systematically examined nor is there a generalised recognised framework for analysing it. For a bullish view, see Vetter (1995). For reviews of the scope for home care and better discharge see Marks (1991) and (1995).

As suggested in the text, the scope for substitution may emerge from a detailed analysis of different ways of providing specific services. One commonly used approach, pathway analysis, is described in Frantz (1994), Jones and Mullikin (1994) and Campuano (1995).

The question of appropriateness is analysed in Hopkins *et al* (1993)and material on variations in intervention rates between geographical areas can be found in MacPherson (1981) and Ham (1988).

Chapter 10

This chapter pays relatively little attention to developments in medical technology since the field has been extensively and intensively surveyed by others. In addition to Schwartz (1994), see Banta (1990), Rawlinson Kelly Whittlestone (1992) and Stocking (1992), all of which go into more detail than is set out in this chapter, though without reaching greater precision on the implications of the developments foreseen. The office of Science and Technology programme entitled *Technology Foresight* includes Health and Life Sciences as one of 15 sectors it revises.

Medical staffing and the role of consultants in particular is the subject of a series of articles in the *British Medical Journal (*1995) entitled 'Rethinking Consultants' starting with Bailey (1995) while the Report of the Medical Workforce Standing Advisory Committee (1955) contains more relevant material.

For a review of the scope for using IT to develop new forms of service, see Gott (1995).

Chapter 11

The literature here is sparse but Pencheon (1995) covers some of the ground eg in relation to use of telephone care. As noted above, the London Implementation Group review of children's services comments on the importance of access and the accommodation option. The notion of equity and its different interpretations are set out in Watt and Sheldon (1993): see also Benzeval (1995), Whitelegg (11982), Mohan (1987).

Chapter 12

Even though the potential and indeed the need for change emerges at several points in this report, for reasons set out in this chapter the overall conclusions are tentative. Others have been more radical: see for example NAHAT (1993) and Vetter (1995), both of which support the case for a small number of centres providing very specialised services and a large number of smaller institutions providing local services. Warner and Riley (1994) also support this pattern of provision but suggest that the district general hospital will take a long time to disappear.

Bibliography

B Abel-Smith (1964), *The Hospitals 1800-1948*, Heinemann, London.

LH Aitken and WS Sage (1993), 'Staffing National Health Care Reforms: a role for advanced practice nurses', *Akron Law Review*, 26, pp 187-211.

DE Allen (1976), *A Short History of the Hospital Service in England and Wales*, Manchester Business School and Centre for Business Research, Manchester.

DE Allen (1979), *Hospital Planning*, Pitman Medical, Tunbridge Wells.

S Amundsen *et al* (1990), 'Abdominal aortic aneurysms: is there an association between surgical volume, surgical experience, hospital type and operative mortality?', *Acta Chirurgica Scandinavia*, 156, pp 323-327.

ID Anderson *et al* (1988), 'Retrospective study of 1000 deaths from injury in England and Wales', *British Medical Journal*, 296, pp 1303-1308.

P Anderson *et al* (1988), 'Use of hospital beds: a cohort study of admissions to a provincial teaching hospital', *British Medical Journal*, 296, pp 911-912.

Association of Anaesthetists of Great Britain and Ireland (1990), *The High Dependency Unit – acute care in the future*, London.

Association of British Neurologists (1990), *A Policy Statement on the Number and Distribution of Consultants in Adult Neurology*, London.

Association of British Neurologists (1993), *Good Neurological Practice*, London.

Association of Cancer Physicians (1994), *Review of the Pattern of Cancer Services in England and Wales*, Southampton.

Audit Commission (1990), *A Short Cut to Better Services, Day Surgery in England and Wales*, HMSO, London.

Audit Commission (1991), *Measuring Quality: the patient's view of day surgery*, London.

Audit Commission (1992), *Lying in Wait: the use of medical beds in acute hospitals*, HMSO, London.

Audit Commission (1993a), *What seems to be the matter? Communication between hospital and patients*, HMSO, London.

Audit Commission (1993b), *Children First: a study of hospital services*. HMSO, London.

Audit Commission (1995), *The Doctor's Tale*, HMSO, London.

EE Bailey and AF Friedlander (1982), 'Market structure and multi-product industries', *Journal of Economic Literature*, xx, pp 1024-1048.

J Bailey (1995), 'Rethinking Consultants: Time for change in traditional working practices?', *British Medical Journal*, 310, pp 788-9.

JE Baker *et al* (1986), 'Community hospitals in Oxfordshire: their effect on the use of specialist inpatient services', *Journal of Epidemiology & Community Health*, 40, pp 117-120.

D Banta (1990), *Emerging and Future Health Care Technology and the Nature of the Hospital*, Welsh Health Planning Forum, Cardiff.

D Banta and M Bos (1991), 'The relation between quantity and quality with coronary artery bypass graft surgery', *Health Policy*, 18, pp 1-10.

DT Barker (1987), 'A motorised surgery unit for treatment of the handicapped patient', *British Dental Journal*, 6 June, pp 436-7.

JA Barondass (1993), 'The future of generalism', *Annals of Internal Medicine*, 119, pp 153-160.

W Bartlett and J Le Grand (undated), *Costs and Trusts*, School for Advanced Urban Studies, Bristol.

W Bartlett and J Le Grand (1992), *The Impact of NHS Reforms on Hospital Costs*, Studies in Decentralisation and Quasi-Markets 8, School for Advanced Urban Studies, Bristol.

AC Bebbington (1988), 'The expectation of life without disability in England and Wales', *Social Science and Medicine*, 27, pp 321-326.

WA Beck *et al* (1988), 'Evaluation of the "golden period" for wound repair: 204 cases from a Third World emergency department', *Annals of Emergency Medicine*, 17, pp 496-500.

GS Becker (1965), 'A theory of the allocation of time', *Economic Journal*, 75, pp 493-517.

R Beech and J Larkinson (1990)'Estimating the financial savings from maintaining the level of acute services with fewer beds', *International Journal of Health Planning and Management*, 5, pp 89-103.

R Beech *et al* (1990), 'Forecasting change', *Health Service Journal*, 100(5220), pp 1438-40 (27 September).

G Bentham (1986), 'Proximity to hospital and mortality from motor vehicle accidents', *Social Science and Medicine*, 23, pp 1001-26.

G Bentham and R Haynes (1986), 'A raw deal in remoter rural areas', *Family Practitioner Services*, 13, pp 84-87.

M Benzeval (1995), 'Health care for all: how to take equity seriously'. In AJ Harrison (ed) (1995), *Health Care UK 1994/95*, King's Fund, London.

D Birkenshaw (1993), 'Palliative care in the acute setting', *Journal of Advanced Nursing*, 18, pp 1665-1666.

N Black and A Johnston (1990), 'Volume and outcome in hospital care: evidence, explanations and implications', *Health Services Management Research*, 3, pp 108-114.

D Blainey *et al* (1990), 'The cost of acute asthma – how much is preventable?', *Health Trends*, 4, pp 151-153.

Blood (1995), 'ASCO/ASM Recommended criteria for the performance of bone marrow transplantation', 75, p 1209.

S Bloomfield and J W Farquhar (1990), 'Is a specialist paediatric diabetic clinic better?', *Archives of Disease in Childhood*, 65, pp 139-140.

JR Border *et al* (1983), 'Prehospital trauma care – stabilise or scoop and run?', *Journal of Trauma*, 23, 708-11.

A Bowling *et al* (1994), 'Who are the consistently high users of health and social services? A follow-up study two and a half years later of people age 85+ at baseline', *Health & Social Care*, 1, pp 277-287

S Boyle and AJ Harrison (1995), 'Provider Competition: Wheel and deal', *Health Service Journal*, 30 March, pp 24-26.

S Brearley (1992), 'Manpower', *British Medical Journal*, 304, pp 832-4.

British Association for Accident and Emergency Medicine (1992), *The Way Ahead*, Royal College of Surgeons, London.

British Association for Paediatric Nephrology (1995), *The Provision of Services in the United Kingdom for Children and Adolescents with Renal Disease*, British Paediatric Association, London.

British Association of Dermatologists (undated), *Dermatology in Practice*.

British Association of Otolaryngologists (1993), *Minimum Requirements for Otolaryngologiy Departments in NHS Hospitals*, London.

British Association of Plastic Surgeons (undated), *Plastic Surgery in the British Isles: a plan for the rest of the 1990s*, London.

British Association of Plastic Surgeons (1994), *Plastic Surgery in the British Isles: present and Future*, London.

British Association of Surgical Oncology (1994), personal communication.

British Association of Urological Surgeons (1993), *The Provision of Urological Services in the UK*, London.

British Cardiac Society (1993), *Strategic Planning for Cardiac Services and the Internal Market*, London.

British Cardiac Society (1994), 'A report of a working group of the British Cardiac Society: cardiology in the district hospital', *British Heart Journal*, 72, pp 303 -308.

British Orthopaedic Association (1992), *The Management of Skeletal Trauma in the United Kingdom*, London.

British Orthopaedic Association and British Association of Plastic Surgeons (1993), *The Early Management of Severe Tibial Fractures: The Need for Combined Plastic and Orthopaedic Management*, London.

British Paediatric Association (1993a), *Hospital Paediatric Medical Staffing*, London.

British Paediatric Association (1993b), *Transfer of Infants and Children for Surgery*, London.

British Paediatric Association (1994), *Purchasers Guide to Paediatrics*, London.

British Society of Gastroenterology (1990), *Provision of Gastrointestinal Endoscopy and Related Services for a District General Hospital*, London.

British Society of Haemotology (1992), *Consultant Haemotology Staffing in the United Kingdom*.

British Thoracic Society (undated), *Manpower Survey*, London.

H Brodsky and A S Hakkert (1983), 'Highway fatal accidents and accessibility of emergency medical services', *Social Science and Medicine*, 17, pp 731-740.

JM Bronstein and MA Morrissey (1990), 'Determinants of rural travel distance for obstetrics care', *Medical Care*, 28, p 853-865.

RH Brook (1994), 'Appropriateness: the next frontier', *British Medical Journal*, 308 pp 218-219.

CE Bucknall *et al* (1988), 'Differences in Hospital Asthma Management', *Lancet,* pp 748-50

LR Burns and DR Wholey (1991), 'The effects of patient, hospital and physician characteristics on length of stay and mortality', *Medical Care*, 29, pp 251-270.

JRG Butler (1995), *Hospital Cost Analysis*, Kluwer, London

K Calman (1993), *Hospital Doctors: training for the future*, Department of Health, London.

R Campbell and A Macfarlane (1995), *Where to be Born? The debate and the evidence*, National Perinatal Epidemiological Unit, Oxford.

EA Campling *et al* (1993), *Report of the National Confidential Enquiry into Peri-operative Deaths 1991/92*, Royal College of Surgeons, London.

TA Campuano (1995), 'Clinical pathways: practical approaches, positive outcomes', *Nursing Management*, 26, pp 34-7.

M Cara (1991), 'Urgences extra-hospitalières', *Bulletin de l'Academie Nationale de Medicine*, 3, pp 351-361.

WJ Carr and PJ Feldstein (1967), 'The relationship of cost to hospital size', *Inquiry*, 4, pp 45-65.

V Carstairs and R Morris (1991), *Deprivation and Health in Scotland*, Aberdeen University Press, Aberdeen.

A Cartwright (1991), 'Changes in life and care in the year before death, 1969-1987', *Journal of Public Health Medicine*, [edition], pp 81-7.

A Cartwright and J Windsor (1992), *Outpatients and Their Doctors: a study of patients, potential patients, general practitioners and hospital doctors*, HMSO, London.

E Catherwood and DJ O'Rourke (1994), 'Critical Pathway Management of Unstable Angina', *Progress in Cardiovascular Diseases*, XXXVII, pp 121-148.

D Chamberlain *et al* (1994), 'Eighth survey of staffing in cardiology in the United Kingdom 1992', *British Heart Journal*, 71, pp 492-500

Clinical Standards Advisory Group (1993), *Access and Availability of Coronary Artery Bypass Graft and Coronary Angioplasty,* HMSO, London.

Clinical Standards Advisory Group (1995), *Urgent and Emergency Admissions to Hospital*, HMSO, London.

RM Coffey (1983), 'The effect of time price on the demand for medical care services', *Journal of Human Resources*, 18, pp 407-424.

P Cohen (1993), 'In search of lost time', *Health Service Journal*, 2 December, p16.

College of Ophthalmologists (1993), *Hospital Eye Service*, London.

P Corris *et al* (1993), *Requirements for Good Practice in Respiratory Medicine*, British Thoracic Society, London.

A Coulter *et al* (1993), 'Diagnostic dilation and curettage: is it used appropriately?' *British Medical Journal*, 306, pp 236-9.

GDM Court (1976), *Fit for the future: the report of the Committee on child health services*, HMSO, London.

TG Cowing and AG Holtmann (1983), 'Multi-product short-run hospital costs functions: empirical evidence and policy implications from cross-section data', *Southern Economic Journal*, 49, pp 637-653.

TG Cowing *et al* (1983), 'Hospital Cost Analysis, Advances in Health Economics and Health Services Research', 4, pp 257-303.

J Cromwell *et al* (1990), 'Learning by doing in CABG surgery', *Medical Care*, 28, pp 6-18.

JG Cullis *et al* (1981), *The Economics of Outpatient Clinic Location: the paediatrics case*, Gower, Farnborough.

A Cuschieri (1993), *Minimal Access Surgery*, HMSO, Edinburgh.

P Cutler (1993), 'Trends in the structure, productivity, effectiveness and unit costs of the hospital and community health services workforce in England: 1971-1991', *Health Economics*, 2, pp 65-75.

J Dale (1992), *Primary Care in A&E: establishing the service*, King's College School of Medicine and Dentistry, London.

JE Daly and PRS Thomas (1992), 'Trauma deaths in the South West Thames region', *Injury*, 6, pp 393-396.

G Davidson (1990), 'Does inappropriate use explain small-area variations in the use of health care services: a critique', *Health Services Research*, 28, 4 pp 389-400

DA Dayhoff and J Cromwell (1993), 'Measuring differences and similarities in hospital caseloads: a conceptual and empirical analysis', *Health Services Research*, 28, pp 293-312.

Department of Health and Social Security (1974), *Community Hospitals: their role and development in the National Health Service*, DHSS, London.

Department of Health and Social Security (1975), *Review of Health Services and Resources: Planning Tasks for 1975/76*, DS 85/75, HMSO, London.

Department of Health and Social Security (1976), *Priorities for Health and Personal Social Services*, HMSO, London.

Department of Health and Social Security (1977), *The Way Ahead*, HMSO, London.

Department of Health and Social Security (1980), *Hospital Services: The Future of Hospital Provision*, HMSO, London.

Department of Health and Social Security (1981a), *Care in Action: a handbook of policies and priorities for the health and personal social services in England*, HMSO, London.

Department of Health and Social Security (1981b), *Report of a Study of the Acute Hospital Sector*, HMSO, London.

Department of Health (1991), *The Welfare of Children and Young People in Hospital*, HMSO, London.

Department of Health (1993a), *Changing Childbirth: report of the expert committee*, HMSO, London.

Department of Health (1993b), *Hospital Doctors: Training for the Future* (Calman Report), HMSO, London.

Department of Health (1993c). Managing the New NHS: functions and responsibilities in the new NHS, HMSO, London

Department of Health Estates Directorate (1989), *Running Costs of Nucleus Hospitals*, London.

Department of Health and Social Security/Welsh Office (1969), *The Functions of the District General Hospital*, Bonham-Carter Committee, HMSO, London.

DHSS Operational Research Section (undated), *Consequences of Size of New District Hospitals*, London.

L Dillner (1993), 'Senior House Officers: the lost tribe', *British Medical Journal*, 307, pp 1549-51

P Dixon *et al*. (1992), *Hospital Services for the 21st Century*, Oxford Regional Health Authority, Oxford.

WH Donovan et al (1984), 'Incidence of medical complications in spinal cord injury: patients in specialised compared with non-specialised centres', *Paraplegia*, 22, pp 283-29.

R Dowie (1989-1991), *Patterns of Medical Staffing: General Medicine, General Surgery, Obstetrics and Gynaecology, Trauma and Orthopaedic Surgery, Ophthalmology, Paediatrics, General Psychiatry Overview*, King's Fund, London.

S Dowling et al (1995), 'With nurse practitioners, who needs house officers?', *British Medical Journal*, 311, pp 309-313.

N Drummond et al (1994), 'Integrated care for asthma: a clinical, social and economic evaluation', *British Medical Journal*, 308, pp 559-564.

JH Duff (1992), 'Specialism and generalism in the future of general surgery', *Canadian Journal of Surgery*, 35 pp 131-135.

J Dukes and R Stewart (1993), 'The use of protocols - a problem', *Advanced Hospital Management*, pp 5-8.

RJ Dunlop et al (1989), 'Preferred versus actual place of death: a hospital palliative care support team experience', *Palliative Medicine*, 3, pp 197-201.

DL Dunn et al (1995), 'Economies of scope in physicians' work: the performance of multiple surgery', *Inquiry*, 32, pp 87-101.

LIA Durojaiye et al (1989), 'Improved primary care: prevent the admission of children to hospital', *Public Health*, 103, pp 181-188.

The Economist (1994a), *Chronicle of a disease foretold*, 22 January, pp 81-2

The Economist (1994b), *The Future of Medicine*, 19 March.

The Economist (1994c), *A heart-warming sort of place*, 29 October, p 73.

N Edwards and V Warneke (1994), 'In the fast lane', *Health Service Journal*, 8 December, pp 30-32.

CV Egleston *et al* (1994), 'Use of a telephone advice line in an accident and emergency department', *British Medical Journal*, 308, p 31.

J Ehrenwerth *et al* (1986), 'Transport of critically ill adults', *Critical Care Medicine*, 14, pp 543-54.

RG Evans (1971), "Behavioural' cost functions for hospitals', *Canadian Journal of Economics*, 4, pp 198-215.

RG Evans (1984), *Strained Mercy: the economics of Canadian health care*, Butterworths, Toronto.

RG Evans and HD Wasker (1972), 'Information theory and the analysis of hospital cost structures', *Canadian Journal of Economics*, V, pp 398-418.

Expert Advisory Group on Cancer to Chief Medical Officers of England and Wales, Consultative Document (1994), *A Policy Framework for Commissioning Cancer Services*, Department of Health, London.

DE Farley and RJ Ozminkowski (1992), 'Volume-outcome relations and inhospital mortality: the effect of changes over time', *Medical Care*, 30, pp 77-94.

A Farmer and A Coulter (1990), 'Organisation of care for diabetic patients in general practice: influence on hospital admissions', *British Journal of General Practice*, 40, pp 56-58.

S Farrar (1993), 'NHS reforms and resource management: whither the hospital?', *Health Policy*, 26, pp 93-104.

C Farrell (1993), *Conflict and change: specialist care in London*, King's Fund, London.

MJG Farthing *et al* (1993), 'Nature and standards of gastrointestinal and liver services in the United Kingdom', *Gut*, 34, pp 1728-1739.

JA Ferguson *et al* (1991a), 'Audit of workload in gynaecology: analysis of time trends from linked statistics', *British Journal of Obstetrics and Gynaecology*, 98, pp 772-777

JA Ferguson *et al* (1991b), 'Workload trends in otolaryngology, some statistical observations from medical record linkage', *Clinical Otolaryngology*, 16, pp 393-398

JA Ferguson *et al* (1991c), 'Ophthalmology in the Oxford Region: analysis of time trends from linked statistics', *Eye*, 5, 379-384

AB Flood *et al* (1984a), 'Does practice make perfect? Part I: The relationship between hospital volume and outcome for selected diagnostic categories', *Medical Care*, 22, pp 98-114.

AB Flood *et al* (1984b), 'Does practice make perfect? Part II: The relation between volume and outcome and other hospital characteristics', *Medical Care*, 22, pp 940-959.

AB Flood and W Scott (1987), *Hospital Structure and Performance*, Johns Hopkins University Press, Baltimore.

DM Fox (1986), *Health Policies, Health Politics*, Princeton, New Jersey.

A Frantz (1994), 'The cardiac care step-down unit at home', *Caring Magazine*, 13, pp 42-48.

MS Freeland (1987), 'Selective contracting for hospital care based on volume, quality and prices: prospects, problems and unanswered questions', *Journal of Health Politics, Policy and Law*, 12, pp 409-426.

N Freemantle *et al* (1992), *The treatment of persistence of glue ear*, Effective Health Care 4, School of Public Health, University of Leeds.

N Freemantle *et al* (1994), *Implementing Clinical Practice Guidelines*, Effective Health Care 8, Nuffield Institute of Health, University of Leeds.

J Frenk (1985), 'The concept and measurement of accessibility', in KL White (ed) (1992), *Health Services Research: An Anthology*, Pan-American Health Organisation, Washington DC.

JF Fries (1980), 'Aging, Natural Death and the Compression of Morbidity', *New England Journal of Medicine*, 303, pp 130-135.
JF Fries (1989), 'The compression of morbidity: near or far?', *Milbank Quarterly*, 67, pp 208-232.

JF Fries *et al* (1993), 'Reducing health care costs by reducing the need and demand for medical services', *New England Journal of Medicine*, 329, 5, pp 321-325.

A Fromet (1979) 'Comparaison des hypertendus hospitalises et consultants dans une unite specialisee', *Achives des Maladies du Coeur et des Vaisseaux*, 72, pp 1137-45.

J Fry and J Horder (1994), *Primary Care in an International Context*, Nuffield Provincial Hospital Trust, London.

AM Garber *et al* (1984), 'Case mix, costs and outcomes', *The New England Journal of Medicine*, 310, pp 1231-1237.

L Garrett (1994), *The Coming Plague: newly emerging diseases in a world out of balance*, Farrer, Strauss and Givoos, New York

D Gentleman and B Jennett (1990), 'Audit of transfer of unconscious head-injured patients', *Lancet*, 335, pp 330-34.

T Geradi (1994), 'A regional hospital association's approach to clinical pathway development', *Journal of Healthcare Policy*, 16, pp 10-14.

AS Gervin and RP Fischer (1982), 'The importance of prompt transport in salvage of patients with penetrating heart wounds', *Journal of Trauma*, 22, pp 443-8.

MJ Goldacre *et al* (1988), 'Trends in episode based and person based rates of admission to hospital in the Oxford record linkage study area', *British Medical Journal*, 296, pp 583-5.

M Gott (1995) *Telematics for Health: the role of telehealth and telemedicine in homes and communities*, Radcliffe Medical Press, Oxford.

TW Grannemann and RS Brown (1986), 'Estimating Hospital Costs: a multiple output analysis', *Journal of Health Economics*, 5, pp 107-127

L Granshaw (1992), 'The rise of the modern hospital in Britain', in A Wear (ed), *Medicine in Society*, Cambridge University Press.

AM Gray (1991), 'A mixed economy of health care: Britain's health service sector in the inter-war period', in A McGuire *et al* (1991), *Providing Health Care: the economics of alternative systems of finance and delivery*, Oxford University Press.

AM Gray and R Steele (1981), 'The economies of specialist and general practitioner units', *Journal of the Royal College of General Practitioners*, 31, pp 586-592.

K Green (1992), *Impact of Advances in Medical Technology on Shifting the Professional and Organisational Boundaries of Health Services,* (unpublished).

R Greenhalgh (1994), 'Commentary: The obituary of general surgery?', *British Medical Journal*, 309, p 388.

AL Greer (1987), 'Rationing Medical Technology: hospital decision making in the United States and England', *International Journal of Technology in Health Care*, 3, pp 199-222.

J Grimley Evans (1993), 'This patient or that patient', in R Smith (ed), *Rationing in Action,* British Medical Journal Press, London.

Gut (1989), 'Staffing of a combined general medical service and gastroenterology unit in a district general hospital', 30, pp 546-550.

C Ham (1981), *Policy-Making in the National Health Service*, Macmillan, London.

C Ham (1982), *Health Policy in Britain*, Macmillan, London.

C Ham (ed) (1988), *Health Care Variations: assessing the evidence*, King's Fund Institute, London.

EL Hannan *et al* (1991), 'Coronary Artery Bypass Surgery: the relationship between inhospital mortality rate and surgical volume after controlling for clinical risk factors', *Medical Care*, 29, pp 1094-1107.

EL Hannan *et al* (1992), 'A longitudinal analysis of the relationship between inhospital mortality in New York State and the volume of abdominal aortic aneurysms of surgeries performed', *Health Services Research*, 27, pp ?-540.

M Harding *et al* (1993), 'Management of malignant teretoma: does referral to a specialist unit matter?', *Lancet* 341, pp 999-1002.

AJ Harrison and J Gretton (1984), *Health Care UK 1984,* Policy Journals, Hermitage.

AJ Harrison and S Prentice (1993), 'Changing boundaries between hospital and community: paediatric and maternity services', in AJ Harrison (ed), *Health Care UK 1992/93*, King's Fund, London.

AJ Harrison *et al* (1995), *Analysing changes in emergency medical admissions*, NHS Trust Federation, London.

AJ Harrison (1996), 'Structural change in hospitals: the implications for research', *Journal of Health Services Research & Policy* (forthcoming).

B Haward (1994), 'Caring for Cancer', *Health Service Journal,* 11 August, pp 22-24.

RM Haynes and CG Bentham (1979), *Community Hospitals and Rural Accessibility*, Saxon House, Farnborough.

RM Haynes and CG Bentham (1982), 'The Effects of Accessibility on General Practitioner Consultations, Outpatient Attendances and Inpatient Admissions in Norfolk, England', *Social Science and Medicine*, 16, pp 561-569.

Health Care Evaluation Unit (1992a), *Hernia Repair: Epidemiologically Based Needs Assessment*, University of Bristol, Bristol.

Health Care Evaluation Unit (1992b), *Cataract Surgery*, University of Bristol, Bristol.

Health and Community Care Research Unit (1995), *Study of Emergency Medical Admissions at Aintree: summary of results*, Liverpool.

AW Heinemann *et al* (1989), 'Functional outcome following spinal cord injury', *Archives of Neurology*, 46, pp 1098-1102.

J Henderson *et al* (1989), 'Use of medical record linkage to study readmission rates', *British Medical Journal*, 299, pp 709–713.

D Hennessy and S Tomlinson (1994), 'The new NHS: challenges and opportunities for medical and nursing education', *Health Trends,* 26, pp 7-10.

J Higgins (1993), *The Future of Small Hospitals in Britain*, University of Southampton.

SD Hillson *et al* (1992), 'Economies of scope and payment for physician services', *Medical Care*, September, 30, pp 822-831.

C Hogg (1992), *Centering Excellence? National and regional health services in London*, King's Fund, London.

A Hopkins *et al* (1993), 'What do we mean by appropriate health care?, *Quality in Health Care*, 2, pp 117-123.

RD Horner *et al* (1995), 'Relationship between physician specialty and the selection and outcome of ischemic stroke patients', *Health Services Research*, 30, pp 279-291.

R Horton (1995), 'Infection: the global threat', *The New York Review of Books*, 6 April, pp 24-217.

House of Commons Committee of Public Accounts (1992), *NHS Accident and Emergency Departments in Scotland*, HMSO, London.

House of Commons Health Committee (1992), *Maternity Care*, HMSO, London.

House of Commons Welsh Affairs Committee (1994), *The use of treatment centres*, HMSO, London.

GP Howell *et al* (1990), 'Long distance travel for routine elective surgery: questionnaire survey of patients' attitudes', *British Medical Journal,* 300, pp 1171-3

S Howelly (1995), 'Reshaping accident and emergency services', *Community Care Management and Planning*, 3, pp 90-95.

D Hughes and D Allen (1993) *Inside the Black Box: obstacles to change in the modern hospital*, unpublished.

J Hughes and P Gordon (1992), *An Optimal Balance*, King's Fund, London.

BT Jackson (1988), 'Whither general surgery?', *Annals of the Royal College of Surgeons England*, 70, p 12.

Joint Cardiology Committee of the Royal College of Physicians of London and the Royal College of Surgeons of England (1992), 'Fourth Report', *British Heart Journal*, 67, pp 106-116.

J Jones *et al* (1993), 'Measuring hospital workload in general medicine', *Health Services Management Research*, pp 156-166.

R Jones *et al* (1988), 'This role of community hospitals', *Health Trends*, 20, pp 45–48

RA Jones and CW Mullikin (1994), 'Collaborative Care: Pathways to Quality Outcomes', *Journal of Healthcare Quality*, 16, pp 10-13.

A Joseph and D Phillips (1984), *Accessibility and Utilisation: geographical perspectives on health care delivery*, Harper & Row, London.

KL Kahn *et al* (1988), 'Measuring the clinical appropriateness of the use of a procedure: can we do it?', *Medical Care*, 26, pp 415–422

JF Kasper *et al* (1992), 'Developing shared decision making programmes to improve the quality of health care', *Journal of Quality Improvement, Quality Review Bulletin*, 18, pp 183-196.

JK Kassirer (1994), 'Access to specialty care', *New England Journal of Medicine*, 331 (17), 1151-3.

JV Kelly and FJ Hellinger (1987), 'Heart disease and hospital deaths: an empirical study', *Health Services Research*, 22, pp 367-395.

S Kendrick (1995), 'Emergency Admissions: what is driving the increase?', *Health Service Journal*, 4 May, pp 26-28.

R Klein (1989), *The Politics of the National Health Service*, Longman, London.

Lancet (1995a), 'Who is a surgeon' ... (editorial), Vol 345, No 8591, pp 663-665.

Lancet (1995b), 'Specialisation, centralised treatment and patient care' (editorial), pp 1251-2.

P Langhorne *et al* (1993), 'Do stroke units save lives?', *Lancet*, 342, pp 395-393.

R Langton Hewer and VA Wood (1992) 'Neurology in the United Kingdom II: a study of current neurological services for adults', *Journal of Neurology, Neurosurgery and Psychology*, 55(supp), pp 8-14.

JP Lathrop (1993), *Restructuring Health Care: the patient focused paradigm*, Josey Bass. San Francisco.

B Leese *et al* (1995), *A Stitch in Time? Minor surgery in general practice*, Centre for Health Economics, University of York.

M Leferve (1992), 'Physician volume and obstetric outcome', *Medical Care*, 30, pp 866-871.

CL Leibson *et al* (1992), 'The compression of morbidity hypotheses: promise and pitfalls of using record-linked data bases to assess secular trends in morbidity and mortality', *Milbank Quarterly*, 70, pp 127-154.

J Lewis (1992), ' "Providing consumers", the state and the delivery of health-care service in twentieth century Britain', in A Wear (ed), *Medicine in Society*, Cambridge University Press.

A Liberati *et al* (1985), 'Process and outcome of care for patients with ovarian cancer', *British Medical Journal*, 291, pp 1007-1012.

London Implementation Group (1993a), *Report of an Independent Review of Specialist Services in London: Cardiac*, HMSO, London.

London Implementation Group (1993b), *Report of an Independent Review of Specialist Services in London: Cardiac*, HMSO, London.

London Implementation Group (1993c), *Report of an Independent Review of Specialist Services in London: Plastics and Burns*, HMSO, London.

London Implementation Group (1993d), *Report of an Independent Review of Specialist Services in London: Children*, HMSO, London.

London Implementation Group (1993e), *Report of an Independent Review of Specialist Services in London: Cancer*, HMSO, London.

London Implementation Group (1993f), *Report of an Independent Review of Specialist Services in London: Renal*, HMSO, London.

London Implementation Group (1993g), *Report of an Independent Review of Specialist Services in London: Neurosciences*, HMSO, London.

HS Luft *et al* (1979), 'Should operations be regionalised? *The New England Journal of Medicine*, 301, pp 1364-1369.

HS Luft *et al* (1990a), 'Does Quality Influence Choice of Hospital?', *Journal of the American Medical Association*, 263 21, pp 2899-2906.

HS Luft *et al* (1990b), *Hospital Volume, Physician Volume and Patient Outcomes: assessing the evidence*, Health Administration Press Perspectives, Ann Arbor.

SC Maerki *et al* (1986), 'Selecting categories of patient for regionalisation: implications of the relationship between volumes and outcomes', *Medical Care*, 24, pp 148-158.

A Mahon *et al* (1994), 'Choice of hospital for elective surgery', in R Robinson and J Le Grand (eds), *Evaluating the NHS Reforms*, King's Fund Institute, London.

F Majeed et al (1994), 'Using Patient and General Practice Characteristics to Explain Variation in Cervical Smear Uptake Rates', British Medical Journal, 308, pp 1272–6

LA Malcolm (1989), 'Decentralisation trends in the management of New Zealand's health services', *Health Policy*, 12, pp 285-299.

LA Malcolm (1990), 'Service Management: New Zealand's model of resource management', *Health Policy*, 16, pp 255-263.

LA Malcolm (1991), 'Service management: a New Zealand model for shifting the balance from hospital to community care', *International Journal of Health Planning and Management*, 6, pp 23-35.

LA Malcolm (1994a),'Primary health care and the hospital and the limits to purchasing', *British Medical Journal*, 310, pp 101-103.

LA Malcolm (1994b), 'Primary Health Care and the Hospital: incompatible organisational concepts?', *Social Science and Medicine*, 39, pp 455-458.

LA Malcolm and P Barnett (1994), 'New Zealand's health providers in an emerging market, *Health Policy*, 29, pp 85-100.

Management Executive, NHS in Scotland (1994a), *Trends in the Use of Acute Beds and the Elderly*, HMSO, London.

Management Executive, NHS in Scotland (1994b), *The Interface between Geriatric Medicine and General Medicine*, HMSO, London.

KG Manton (1982), 'Changing concepts of morbidity and mortality in the elderly population', *Milbank Memorial Fund Quarterly*, 60, pp 183-244.

KG Manton (1991), 'The dynamics of population aging: demography and policy analysis', *Milbank Quarterly*, 69, pp 309-338.

L Marks (1991), *Home and Hospital Care: Redrawing the boundaries*, King's Fund Institute, London.

L Marks (1994), *Seamless Care or Patchwork Quilt: discharging patients from acute hospital care*, King's Fund Institute, London.

S Martin and P Smith (1995), *Modelling Waiting Times for Elective Surgery*, Centre for Health Economics, University of York.

JD Mayer (1979a), 'Emergency medical services: delays, response time and survival', *Medical Care*, XVII, pp 818-827.

JD Mayer (1979b), 'Seattle's Paramedic Programme: Geographical Distribution, Response Time and Mortality', *Social Science and Medicine*, 13D, pp 45-51.

JD Mayer (1979c), 'Paramedic Response Time and Survival from Cardiac Arrest', *Social Science and Medicine*, 13D, pp 267-271.

A Maynard and A Walker (1993), *Planning the Medical Workforce: struggling out of the time warp*, Centre for Health Economics, University of York, Discussion Paper 105.

A Maynard and A Walker (1995), 'Managing the medical workforce: time for improvements?', *Health Policy*, 31, pp 1-16.

CS McArdle and D Hole (1991), 'Impact of variability among surgeons on postoperative morbidity and mortality and ultimate survival', *British Medical Journal*, 302, pp 1501-7.

A McGuire *et al* (1988), The economics of health care: an introductory text, RKP, London.

M McGurk and FW Porrell (1984), 'Spatial Patterns of Hospital Utilization: the impact of distance and time', *Inquiry*, Spring, pp 84-95.

M McKee and N Black (1991), 'Hours of work of junior hospital doctors: is there a solution?', *Journal of Management in Medicine*, 5:3, pp 40-54.

M McKee and A Clarke (1995), 'Guidelines, enthusiasms, uncertainty, incompatible organisational concepts? *Social Science and Medicine*, 39, pp 455-458.

T McKeown (1965), *Medicine in Modern Society*, Allen and Unwin, London.

S McLafferty and D Broe (1990), 'Patient outcomes and regional planning of coronary care services: a location allocation approach', *Social Science and Medicine*, 30, pp 297-304.

BP McNicholl *et al* (1993), 'Transatlantic perspectives of trauma systems', *British Journal of Surgery*, 80, pp 985-986.

BP McNicholl (1994), 'The golden hour and prehospital trauma care', *Injury*, 25, pp 251-254.

K McPherson *et al* (1981), 'Regional variations in the use of common surgical procedures: within and between England and Wales, Canada and the United States of America', *Social Science and Medicine*, 15A, pp 273-288.

Medical Workforce Standing Advisory Committee: second report (1995), *Planning the Medical Workforce*, Department of Health, London.

PC Merry (1990), 'Day surgery: a neglected opportunity' in Harrison AJ (ed), *Health Care* UK 1990, Ppolicy Journals, Hermitage.

A Metcalf and K McPherson (1995), *Study of Provision of Intensive Care in England 1993*, London School of Hygiene & Tropical Medicine, London.

JA Michaels *et al* (1994), 'Organisation of vascular surgical services: evolution or revolution?', *British Medical Journal*, 309, pp 387-8.

RG Milne (1993), 'Contractors' experience of compulsory competitive tendering: a case study of contract cleaners in the NHS', *Public Administration*, 71, pp 301-321.

RG Milne and M McGee (1992), 'Compulsory competitive tendering in the NHS: a new look at some old estimates', *Fiscal Studies*, 13:3, pp 96-111.

Ministry of Health (1959), The Welfare of Children in Hospital (The Platt Report), HMSO, London.

Ministry of Health (1962), *Hospital Plan for England and Wales*, Cmnd 1604, HMSO, London.

Ministry of Health (1966), *The Hospital Building Programme; A Revision of the Hospital Plan for England and Wales*, Cmnd 3000, HMSO, London.

Ministry of Health (1969), *The Functions of the District General Hospital*, HMSO, London.

Ministry of Health and Social Services (1965), *Hospital Plan for Northern Ireland 1966-75*, Cmd 497, HMSO.

AJ Mohan (1992), 'Who foots the bill?', *Health Service Journal,* 27 August, pp 22-3.

GT Moore (1992), 'The case of the disappearing generalist: does it need to be solved?' *Milbank Quarterly*, 70, pp 361-379.

RC Morey *et al* (1992), 'The trade-off between hospital cost and quality of care, *Medical Care*, 30, pp 677-695.

DC Morrell *et al* (1993), *Five Essays on Emergency Pathways*, King's Fund Institute, London.

RL Morrill *et al* (1970), 'Factors influencing distances travelled to hospital', *Economic Geography*, 46, pp 161-171.

F Moss and M McNichol (1995), 'Alternative models of organisation are needed', *British Medical Journal*, 310, pp 925-928.

M Mugford (1990), 'Economies of scale and low risk maternity care', *Maternity Action*, pp 6-8.

E Munoz *et al* (1990a), 'Economies of scale, physician volume for neurosurgery patients and the diagnostic related group prospective payment system', *Neurosurgery*, 26, pp 156-161.

E Munoz *et al* (1990b), 'Economies of scale, physician volume for urology patients and the DRG prospective hospital payment system', *Urology*, XXXVI, pp 471-476.

E Munoz *et al* (1990c), 'Costs, quality and the volume of surgical oncology procedures', *Archives of Surgery*, 125, pp 360-368.

E Munoz *et al* (1990d), 'Economic of scales, physician volume for orthopedic surgical patients and the DRG prospective payments system', *Orthopedics*, 13, pp 39-44.

E Murphy (1993), 'Changing Boundaries between Hospital and Community: services for elderly people', in A Harrison (ed), *Health Care UK 1992/93*, Policy Journals.

MVA Consulting (1987), *The Value of Travel Time Savings*, Policy Journals, Hermitage.

NAHAT (1993), *Re-inventing Health Care*, NAHAT, Birmingham.

NAHAT (1995), *Acting on the Evidence*, NAHAT, Birmingham.

National Audit Office (1987), *Competitive Tendering for Support Services in the National Health Service*, HMSO, London.

National Audit Office (1990), *National Health Service: Patient Transport Services*, HMSO, London.

National Audit Office (1992), *Accident and Emergency Departments in England*, HMSO, London.

National Audit Office (1995), *Contracting for Acute Health Care in England*, HMSO, London. RM Nesse and GC Williams (1995), *Evolution and Healing*, Weidenfeld and Nicholson, London.

New England Journal of Medicine Editorial (1994), 'Access to Specialty Care', 331, pp 1151-1152.

NHS Centre for Research and Dissemination (1995a), *Which way forward for the care of critically ill children?*, CRD Report 1, University of York.

NHS Centre for Research and Dissemination (1995b), *Relationship between Volume and Quality of Health Care: A review of the literature*, CRD Report 2, University of York.

NHS Executive Anglia and Oxford Region (1995a), *Opportunities in Emergency Health Care*, Milton Keynes.

NHS Executive Anglia and Oxford Region (1995b), *Emergency Care Handbook*, Milton Keynes.

NHS Executive South Thames (undated), *Journeys into the Unknown*, Bexley.

NHS Executive (1994), *The Patient's Progress: towards a better service*, HMSO, London.

NHS Management Executive (1991), *Day surgery: making it happen*, HMSO, London.

NHS Management Executive (1992), *Patient Hotels: a quality alternative to ward care*, HMSO, London.

NHS Management Executive (1993), *Contracting for Specialised Services: a practical guide*, Leeds.

NHS Management Executive (1994a), *Medical Staffing Policies: a time for change*, Leeds.

NHS Management Executive (1994b), *The Operation of the NHS Internal Market*, Leeds.

JP Nicholl *et al* (1994), 'A comparison of the costs and performance of an emergency helicopter and land ambulances in a rural area', *Injury*, 25, pp 145-153.

Office of Science and Technology (1995), Technology Foresight: health and life sciences, HMSO, London.

Office of Technology Assessment (1987), *Rural Emergency Medical Services*, US Government Printing Office, Washington.

Office of Technology Assessment (1988), *The Quality of Medical Care: information for consumers*, US Government Printing Office, Washington.

LJ Opit *et al* (1991), 'Use of operating theatres: the effect of case-mix and training in general surgery', *Annals of the Royal College of Surgeons of England*, 73, pp 389-393

LM Osman *et al* (1994), 'Reducing hospital admission through computer supported education for asthma patients', *British Medical Journal*, 304, pp 568-71.

T Packwood *et al* (1991), *Hospitals in Transition: the resource management experiment*, Open University Press, Milton Keynes.

D Parkin and J Henderson (1985), *Estimating the Cost of Patients' and Visitors' Travel to Hospital,* Health Economics Research Unit, University of Aberdeen.

RE Peak (1990), 'Does inappropriate use explain small-area variations in the use of health services? a reply', *Health Services Research*, 28, pp 400-418

M Pearson (1992), 'Outpatients Outclassed', *Health Service Journal*, 15 October, pp 28-29

MG Pearson *et al* (1995), 'National audit of acute severe asthma in adults admitted to hospital', *Quality in Health Care*, 4, pp 24-30.

D Pencheon (1995), *Review of the Published Evidence: What the literature says*, NHS Executive Anglia and Oxford Region, Milton Keynes.

PE Pepe *et al* (1987), 'The relationship between total prehospital time and outcome in hypotensive victims of penetrating injuries', *Annals of Emergency Medicine*, 16, pp 293-7.

JC Petrie *et al* (1989), *Computer-assisted shared care: the Aberdeen Blood Pressure clinic*, *Journal of Hypertension*, 7(supp3), pp 103-108.

CS Phibbs *et al* (1993), 'Choice of hospital for delivery: a comparison of high risk and low risk women', *Health Services Research*, 28, pp 202-222.

MM Pollack *et al* (1991), 'Improved outcomes from tertiary center pediatric intensive care: a statewide comparison of tertiary and nontertiary care facilities', *Critical Care Medicine*, 19, pp 150-159.

S Ramaiah (1994), 'Community hospitals in the NHS', *British Medical Journal*, 308, pp 487-88

Rawlinson, Kelly, Whittlestone (1991), *Trends in health building developments 1965-1990*, RKW, London.

Rawlinson, Kelly, Whittlestone (1992), *The Shape of Things to Come*, RKW, London.

Rawlinson, Kelly, Whittlestone (1993), *Patient Focused Care: a suitable case for treatment?*, RKW, London.

S Read and K Gravon (1994), *Reduction of Junior Doctors' Hours in Trent Region: the nursing contribution*, University of Sheffield, Centre for Health and Related Research.

A Redmond *et al.* (1993), 'A trauma centre in the UK', *Annals of the Royal College of Surgeons*, 75, pp 317-320.

GJG. Rees *et al* (1991), 'Clinical oncology services to district general hospitals', *Clinical Oncology*, 3, pp 41-45.

J Rees (1995), 'Rethinking Consultants: Where medical science and human behaviour meet', *British Medical Journal*, 310, pp 850-3.

N Reid and C Todd (1989), 'Travel to hospital', *Health Services Management*, June, pp 129-133.

Renal Association (1991), *Provision of Services for Adult Patients with Renal Disease in the United Kingdom*, London.

Report of the Inquiry into London's Health Service, *Medical Education and Research* (Tomlinson Report), 1992, HMSO.

Report to the Royal College of Physicians (London) Gastroenterology Committee and the Clinical Services Committee of the British Society of Gastroenterology (1989), 'Staffing of a combined general medical service and gastroenterology unit in a district general hospital', *Gut*, 30, 546-550.

TC Ricketts and JM Lambrew (1992), *The Future of the Small Rural Hospital*, a policy review for the Milbank Memorial Fund, unpublished.

J Rigby (1978), *Access to Hospitals: a literature review*, Transport and Road Research Laboratory, Bracknell.

C Roberts *et al* (1995), 'Rationing is a desperate measure', *Health Service Journal*, 12 January, p15.

J Roberts (1995), 'Rethinking Consultants: Specialists in the United States: what lessons?', *British Medical Journal*, 310, pp 724-7.

JM Robine *et al* (1992), *Health Expectancy*, HMSO, London.

JC Robinson (1994), 'The changing boundaries of the American hospital', *The Milbank Quarterly*, 72, pp 259-275

JC Robinson (1995), *Institutional Economics, Organisational Innovation and Vertical Integration in Health Care*, Paper given to International Workshop in Health Economics, Paris.

M Roland and A Coulter (1992), *Hospital Referrals*, Oxford University Press, Oxford.

NP Roos *et al* (1993), 'Living longer but doing worse: assessing health status in elderly persons at two points in time in Manitoba, Canada 1971 and 1983', *Social Science and Medicine*, 36, pp 273-282.

NP Roos and D Lyttle (1985), 'The centralisation of operations and access to treatment: total hip replacement in Manitoba', *American Journal of Public Health*, 25, pp 130-133

N Rousseau *et al* (1994), *Primary Health Care in Rural Areas*, Centre for Health Services Research, University of Newcastle-upon-Tyne.

Royal College of Ophthalmologists (1993), *Hospital Eye Service*, London.

Royal College of General Practitioners (1983), *General Practitioner Hospitals*, Exeter.

Royal College of General Practitioners (1990), *Community Hospitals: preparing for the future*, London.

Royal College of Physicians and Royal College of Psychiatrists (1995), *The Psychological Care of Medical Patients*, London.

Royal College of Surgeons of England (1985), *Surgical Services for Small Communities: the role of the general practitioner hospital*, London.

Royal College of Surgeons of England (1986) *Report of the Working Party on Head Injuries*, London.

Royal College of Surgeons of England (1988), *The Management of Patients with Major Injuries*, London.

Royal Commission on the National Health Service (1979), *Royal Commission on the National Health Service: report*, London.

R Rutledge *et al* (1993), 'An analysis of the association of trauma centres with per capita hospitalisation and death rates from injury', *Annals of Surgery*, 218:4, pp 512-524.

S Ryder *et al* (undated), *Measuring clinical need: when do hospital specialties need to be close to one another?*, Centre for Health Economics, University of York.

A Sadler *et al* (1993), 'Specialist practice for minor oral surgery: a comparative audit of third molar surgery', *British Dental Journal*, 174, pp 273-277

JS Sampalis *et al* (1992), 'Standardised Mortality Ratio Analysis on a sample of severely injured patients from a large Canadian city without regionalised trauma care', *Journal of Trauma*, 33, pp 205-212.

H Sanderson *et al* (1995), 'Health care resource group version 2', *Journal of Public Health Medicine*, 17, pp 349–354.

GR Schwartz *et al* (1989), *Emergency Medicine: the essential update*, W B Saunders, London.

WB Schwartz (1994), 'In the pipeline: a work of valuable technology', *Health Affairs*, Summer, pp 71-79.

A Scott (1995), *Primary or Secondary Care? Economics and the interface between primary and secondary care*, Health Economics Research Unit, University of Aberdeen.

A Scott and D Parkin (1994), *Investigating Hospital Efficiency in the New NHS: the role of the cost function*, Health Economics Research Unit, Discussion Paper 05/94, University of Aberdeen, Aberdeen.

Scottish Health Service Advisory Council (1993), *Report of the Working Group on Cardio-Pulmonary Resuscitation*, HMSO, Edinburgh.

Scottish Home and Health Department (1966), *Review of the Hospital Plan for Scotland*, Cmd 2877, HMSO, Edinburgh.

Scottish Office (1992), *Management of Non-Surgical Cancer Services in Scotland*, HMSO, Edinburgh.

Scottish Office (1994), *Emergency Healthcare in Scotland*, HMSO, Edinburgh.

E Scrivens (1994), *Shifting Boundaries: possible futures for primary care*, Centre for the Analysis of Social Policy, University of Bath.

M Sculpher (1993), *A Snip at the Price? A Review of the Economics of Minimal Access Surgery,* Health Economics Research Group Paper No 11, Brunel University.

M Seabrook *et al* (1994), *Widening the Horizons of Medical Education*, Department of General Practice, King's College School of Medicine and Dentistry.

TA Sheldon (1991), 'The NHS Review and the funding of teaching hospitals', *Journal of Management in Medicine*, 5, pp 6-17.

S Shortell and J Logerfo (1981), 'Hospital Medical staff organisation and quality of care: results for myocardial infarction and appendectomy', *Medical Care,* 19, pp 1041-1053.

S Shortell *et al* (1976), 'The effects of management practices on hospital efficiency and quality of care', in S Shortell and N Brown (eds), *Organisational Research in Hospital*, Blue Cross Association.

S Shortell *et al* (1995), 'Reinventing the American hospital', *The Milbank Quarterly*, 73, pp 131-160.

GRM Sichel and DJ Hall (1982), 'The place of general practitioner hospitals in the organisation of hospital services', *Health Trends,* 14, pp 21-23.

K Sikora and J Waxman (1992), Going for cure: a strategy for London's cancer services in the next century, Hammersmith Hospital Dept of Clinical Oncology, London.

FA Sloan *et al* (1989), 'Is there a rationale for regionalising organ transplantation services', *Journal of Health Politics, Policy and Law,* 14, pp 115-165.

RF Smith *et al* (1990), 'The impact of volume on outcome in seriously injured trauma patients: two years experience of the Chicago trauma system', *Journal of Trauma,* 30, pp 1066-1075

Society of British Neurological Surgeons (1993), *Safe Neurosurgery: the maintenance and development of high standards*, London.

BJ Soldo and KG Manton (1985), 'Health status and service needs of the oldest old: current patterns and future trends', *Milbank Memorial Fund Quarterly*, 63, pp 286-319.

J Soper and JJ Jones (1985), 'Cost-effectiveness of surgery in small "local" hospitals', *Community Medicine*, 7, pp 257-264.

South East Thames Regional Health Authority (1991), *Shaping the Future: a review of acute services.*

J Spiby *et al* (1995), Throw out the Bricks, Build the Service, King's Fund, London.

M Sramek *et al* (1994), 'Telephone triage of cardiac emergency calls by dispatchers: a prospective study of 1386 emergency calls', *British Heart Journal,* 71, pp 440-445.

Steering Committee on Future Health Scenarios (1993), *Primary Care and Home Care Scenarios 1990-2005*, Kluwer Academic.

R Stevens (1989), *In Sickness and in Wealth, American Hospitals in the Twentieth Century*, Basic.

M Stewart and LJ Donaldson (1991), 'Travelling for earlier surgical treatment: the patient's view', *British Journal of General Practice*, 41 pp 508-9.

CA Stiller (1988), 'Centralisation of treatment and survival rates for cancer', *Archives of Disease in Childhood*, 63, pp 23-30.

CA Stiller (1994), 'Centralised treatment, entry to trials and survival', *British Journal of Cancer*, 70, pp 352-362.

CA Stiller and GJ Draper (1989), 'Treatment centre size, entry to trials, and survival in acute lymphoblastic leukemia', *Archives of Disease in Childhood*, 4, pp 657-661.

JA Stilwell (1979), 'Relative costs of home and hospital confinement', *British Medical Journal*, pp 257-9.

JA Stilwell (1993), 'Pathology Service', in AJ Harrison (ed) (1993), *Health Care UK 1992/93*, Policy Journals, Hermitage.

JA Stilwell and C Hawley (1991), 'The costs of nursing care', *Journal of Nursing Management*, 1, pp 25-30.

B Stocking (1992), *Medical Advances: the future shape of acute services*, King's Fund, London.

JD Stoeckle (1995), 'The citadel cannot hold', *The Milbank Quarterly*, 73, pp 3- 17.

FM Sullivan and TM Hoare (1990), 'New Referrals to Rheumatology Clinics- Why do they keep coming back?', *British Journal of Rheumatology*, 29, pp 53-57.

JC Sutton (1990), 'Organisation and planning of ambulance transport services in England and Wales', *Transport Reviews*, 10, pp 149-170.

D Teece (1980), 'Economies of scope and the scope of the enterprise', *Journal of Economic Behaviour and organisation*, 1, pp 223-247.

J Templeton (1994), 'Organising the Management of Life-Threatening Injuries', *Journal of Bone and Joint Surgery*, (British Volume), pp. 3-5.

M Tew (1976), *What Do Hospitals Do?* University of Nottingham, Nottingham.

CJ Todd *et al* (1995), 'Differences in mortality after fracture of hip: the East Anglian audit', *British Medical Journal*, 310, pp 904-8.

JW Todd (1987), 'Specialists should also be generalists', *Journal of the Royal Society of Medicine*, 80, p 153-156.

RAR Treasure and JAJ Davies (1990), 'Contribution of a general practitioner hospital: a further study', *British Medical Journal*, 300, pp 644-6.

DD Turnkey (1984), 'Is ALS necessary for pre-hospital trauma care?', *Journal of Trauma*, 24, pp 81-2.

H Tucker (1987), *The Role and Function of Community Hospitals*, King's Fund, London.

UK Health Departments, Joint Consultants Committee and Chairmen of Regional Health Authorities (1987), *Hospital Medical Staffing: achieving a balance.*

University of York Health Economics Consortium (1991), *A New Methodology for Prioritising Capital Schemes*, York.

N Vetter (1995), *The Hospital*, Chapman & Hall, London.

MG Vita (1990), 'Exploring hospital production relationships with flexible functional forms', *Journal of Health Economics*, 9, pp 1-21.

T Waidmann *et al* (1995), 'The illusion of failure: trends in the self-reported health of the US elderly', *Milbank Quarterly*, 73, pp 253-285.

M Warner *et al* (1993), *Blurring the boundaries – the future of hospital and primary care; the case of gastrointestinal disease*, Welsh Health Planning Forum, Cardiff.

M Warner and C Riley (1994), *Closer to Home*, NAHAT, Birmingham.

J Wasson *et al* (1992), 'Telephone care as a substitute for routine clinical follow-up, *Journal of the American Medical Association*, 267, pp 1788-1793.

IS Watt and TA Sheldon (1993), 'Rurality and resource allocation in the UK', *Health Policy,* 26, pp 19-27.

A Wear (ed) (1992), *Medicine in Society*, Cambridge University Press, Cambridge.

WD Weaver *et al* (1988), 'Use of the automatic external defibrillator in the management of out of hospital cardiac arrest', *The New England Journal of Medicine*, 319, pp 661-666.

C Webster (1988), *The Health Service since the War*, HMSO, London.

MA Weingarten (1982), 'Telephone consultation with patients: a brief study and review of the literature', *Journal of the Royal College of General Practitioners*, 32, pp 766-770.

Welsh Consumer Council (1986), *Within Reach of Health Care*, Cardiff.

Welsh Consumer Council (1988), *Getting to Out-patient clinics*, Cardiff.

Welsh Consumer Council (1989), *Better Access: ways to improve access to outpatients clinics*, Cardiff.

Welsh Health Planning Forum (1993), *Health and Social Care 2010*, Cardiff.

Welsh Health Planning Forum (1995), *Getting the Best for Patients: Effectiveness in medical imaging*, Cardiff.

JE Wennberg *et al* (1987), 'Are hospital services rationed in New Haven or over-utilised in Boston?', *Lancet*, pp 1185-9.

JG West (ed) (1983), *Trauma Care Systems*, Praeger, New York.

J Whitelegg (1982), *Inequalities in health care*, Straw Barnes, Retford.

JEA Wickham (1993), 'An introduction to minimally invasive therapy', *Health Policy,* 23, pp 7-15.

JEA Wickham (1994), 'Minimal invasive surgery: future developments', *British Medical Journal,* 308, pp 193-308.

D Wilkin and C Dorner (1990), *General Practitioner Referrals to Hospital*, Centre for Primary Care Research, University of Manchester, Manchester.

RD Willig (1979), 'Multiproduct technology and market structure', *American Economic Review*, 69, pp 346-351

A Witz (1992), *Professions and Patriarchy*, Routledge, London.

John R Woods *et al* (1992), 'The learning curve and the cost of heart transplantation', *Health Services Research,* 27, pp 219-238.

DW Yates *et al* (1992), 'Preliminary analysis of the care of injured patients in 33 British hospitals – first report of the United Kingdom major trauma study', *British Medical Journal*, 305, pp 737-40.

Index